Positive Psychology and Disability Series

Series Editors
Michael L. Wehmeyer, Beach Center on Disability
University of Kansas
Lawrence, KS, USA

Karrie A. Shogren, Kansas University Center on Developmental Disabilities
University of Kansas
Lawrence, KS, USA

The **Positive Psychology and Disability** book series provides comprehensive coverage of research and practice issues pertaining to the application of constructs and principles from the discipline of positive psychology across the disability context. In addition, books in the series address the application of strengths-based approaches to understanding disability and designing and implementing supports to enable people with disabilities to live, learn, work, and play as meaningful participants in their communities. Drawing from traditional areas of focus in positive psychology, series books:

- Provide cutting-edge research and practice that can improve the quality of life and well-being of people with disabilities.
- Address theory and research across such areas as hope, optimism, self-determination, and character strengths.
- Examine research- and evidence-based practices to promote involvement in goal setting, problem solving, and decision making.
- Synthesize research and practice from multiple disciplines and apply strengths-based approaches to disability.

Volumes published in this series are must-have resources for researchers, professors, clinicians and related professionals, and graduate students in developmental and positive psychology, special education, social work, child and school psychology, and other allied disciplines.

Ryan M. Niemiec • Dan Tomasulo

Character Strengths and Abilities Within Disabilities

Advances in Science and Practice

Springer

Ryan M. Niemiec
VIA Institute on Character
Cincinnati, OH, USA

Dan Tomasulo
Spirituality Mind Body Institute
Teachers College, Columbia University
New York, USA

Positive Psychology and Disability Series
ISBN 978-3-031-36293-4 ISBN 978-3-031-36294-1 (eBook)
https://doi.org/10.1007/978-3-031-36294-1

This Springer imprint is published by the registered company Springer Nature Switzerland AG
The registered company address is: Gewerbestrasse 11, 6330 Cham, Switzerland

For all the people who have not been seen.

Also, for James O. Pawelski:
RMN: During our Aristotelian friendship calls, I told James my second son was born with Down syndrome. I was surprised a couple months later when The Oxford Handbook of Positive Psychology and Disability showed up at my doorstep, unannounced, from him. This creative act of kindness literally catalyzed numerous projects (still going on today, including this book) in the science and practice of character strengths, positively impacting innumerous people.
DT: James is a teacher/mentor, colleague, and friend that has awakened my desire for excellence in writing and authenticity in teaching. He is an exemplar—a philosopher skilled in the art of living. There is something James' former students say about him. It is about his character strengths and approach to teaching. We say of James that he is the only professor we know of who can hug you— and kick you in the butt at the same time. For me this has been especially true, and I am forever grateful.

Preface

All of us, if we live long enough, will experience what can be termed "a disability" in our life. This book is about the human experience. It is about the deep humanity within all of us.

It is really about seeing. It's about seeing people at their core—seeing what's best in people; seeing what is typically unattended to; seeing the ability, the possibility, and the capacity in people.

We've Come a Long Way

Deficit-based. Problem-focused. Dis-abled. These words describe how people with disabilities have largely been perceived or approached over the decades. It is the general mindset that has been taken when someone is perceived as different, abnormal, or somehow "less than." But, there has been a slow awakening over the last couple decades. Practitioners and researchers are beginning to see the strengths in people with disabilities. Organizations, classrooms, parents, counselors, and support staff are referring to themselves as "strengths-based." Positive skills are becoming an important building block, a focal point in helping people. External supports and resources are being developed. Special talents are being highlighted when apparent, and interests/passions are being assessed and encouraged. This wonderful shift is what we refer to as *Strengths-Based: Phase 1*. This is the phase occupied by the majority of organizations, practitioners, and researchers who consider themselves "strengths-based."

This book appreciates this phase and those kinds of strengths and will discuss that work. However, we see a new phase rising. We see new scientific assessments, field studies, and experiments being conducted on another area of strengths in the disability field. That area is arguably the most important category of strengths in human beings, because it's the only category that reflects core identity—who the person is—their best qualities. That area is called character strengths. The education, science, and practice in this area of character strengths is the emerging shift in the disability field, across disabilities and abilities. This is *Strengths-Based: Phase 2*. Therefore, Strengths-Based: Phase 2 will be the focal point of every chapter in this book.

A Word About Disability

The term disability engenders different dialectics in which we can understand and approach it.

We'll be honest with you. A part of us didn't want to use the term "disability" in the title of this book. Another part of us wanted to say it "loud and clear." We believe the essence of both of these can be true, and also be essential throughout this book. Our aim is to emphasize that which is best in human beings and to do that across a wide range of differences in the human experience—differences that can be debilitating, can be life-giving, neither, or both. For many, their diagnosis is not noteworthy, not noticed much in their life nor particularly relevant for their day to day activities. Yet, if we didn't use the term, how would many of the professionals (researchers, academics, students, practitioners), who most crave this material, find the book, or find the material within it?

This is a book that examines the differences in human experiences. These are differences that can be listed in disability categories in all-or-none terms, meaning that one meets particular criteria (e.g., biological, psychological, social) and has the disability or does not meet the criteria and does not have it. In terms of the manifestations and expressions of the disability, we view it on a continuum—this means each behavior or psychological phenomena expresses itself in degrees of more or less; for example, more or less adaptive, more or less attentive. Character strengths are also viewed with this dimensional lens, being expressed along continua of more or less; for example, a person becomes more and more creative in a particular situation and less creative in another. Perhaps this is another dialectic—categories versus dimensions—that we can hold together. There can be truth, insight, and utility in both.

A flaw in becoming locked into over-categorizing disabilities is that a disability can become the sole focus, the default by which everything else filters through. The humanity is stripped away. The uniqueness and individuality are lost. This happens a lot in contemporary society. But, character strengths bring that humanity back. The identification, exploration, encouragement, and actions filled with hope, teamwork, gratitude, perseverance, curiosity, humility, and humor offer a language for that humanity.

The Chapters Layout and Internal Structure

This book emphasizes core concepts, research, and practice on the intersection of character strengths and various disabilities/abilities. The general structure for the book is to flow across three sections, from foundations to specific disabilities to special topics. In Chaps. 1 and 2, we lay the foundations for what is meant by strengths-based and what is meant by character strengths. In Chaps. 3 through 7, we cover a wide range of disabilities and their intersection with character strengths, including intellectual/developmental disability, autism, physical disorders, medical disorders, and various psychological disorders, with specific chapters focused on trauma and also ADHD. The third section of the book focuses on special topic areas relating to intellectual/developmental disabilities. In those chapters, we delve into dual-diagnosis, justice-equity-diversity-inclusion (JEDI), and spirituality/meaning.

Each of the ten chapters contains the following internal structure:

- *Chapter overview*: a brief overview of the chapter's contents and its purpose.
- *The concepts*: the core ideas and areas to know about the chapter's contents.
- *The science*: the main scientific findings to date on the topic or population.
- *The practice*: core practices, practical considerations, and elements of a strengths-based approach for that population or topic area. The focus of this section is on the strongest evidence or strongest base for that evidence which might be theoretical or hypothetical. The emphasis is the application of the science and core concepts.
- *Future directions*: considerations for the science to advance, relating to the content discussed.
- *Key takeaways*: a summary of important points in the chapter.
- *References*: documentation of where previous findings and insights came from as well as an acknowledgment of the wisdom that came before us.

Who This Book Is For

We have written this book to make a positive impact on the following groups:

- *Scholars/academics/researchers*: those aiming to identify new areas of study to have a positive impact, to integrate character strengths into existing/future studies and programs, to conduct new intervention studies, and to advance the science of character strengths with populations in need. This includes professors, scientists, writers, many in academia.
- *Practitioners*: those who aim to help someone with a disability to better integrate character strengths into their mindset, conversations, interventions, programs, supervision, leadership, and system as a whole. This includes social workers, coaches, managers, psychologists, counselors, teachers, medical teams, support teams, and paraprofessionals.
- *Leaders*: those organization leaders, nonprofit innovators and change-makers, policy makers, and governmental/agency leaders who aim to attend to and facilitate character strengths in their organizations and systems as an approach for culture change, leadership development, personal development, and care for the staff and the clients in the system they serve.

- *Students*: Students may fit into one or more of the preceding categories and also warrant their own designation. Students are the future of the field. A foundation in character science, pathways to distill the science into practical applications, and examples of integration to serve various populations is a strong way to bolster one's future work, innovations, and applications.

We are pleased you are on this journey! We welcome you to share with us about your scientific and practical endeavors with this exciting work.

We leave you with this poem about the potential of character strengths, which also reflects many cases and content in this book.

"We See, You See"

We see the nonverbal boy express curious facial expressions and playful humor that disarms and connects with classmates and teachers,

We see the college student, whose learning challenges make her feel she's in a void of uncertainty and confusion, yet she bravely takes on every obstacle, steadfast and strong,

We see the man, steeped in depression, use newfound curiosity to investigate his suffering and creativity to deeply engage himself in different self-care approaches,

We see the woman with Down syndrome give public presentations and use honesty to share her personal struggles and express her hope to inspire others to see the good within themselves,

We see the leader who channels his hyperactivity into inspiring creativity and a kindly zest that unites the many employees of his organization,

We see the mother of three, stunned by her new terminal diagnosis, turns to a mindset of gratitude, teamwork, and love, that models a way forward for her family and community,

And what have you seen?

Have you noticed that there is strength potential in every person in your life?

Have you seen the beauty of your kindness and social intelligence when you have helped someone?

Have you appreciated your love of learning that extends further and further to find new paths for helping others?

Have you seen the power of temperance when connecting with others—that grounding force of humility, the release of forgiveness, the pause brought by prudence, and the artful control of self-regulation?

Have you noticed that in every positive experience you have, there is a character strength that contributes to it?

And in every adversity, there are character strength seeds of growth waiting to be watered?

What do you see? What do *you* see?

Cincinnati, OH, USA Ryan M. Niemiec
New York, NY, USA Dan Tomasulo

Acknowledgments

We offer a humble bow of gratitude to the many people—named and unnamed—who contributed to this book or to our inspiration for it. This includes the positive psychology and disability series editors Mike Wehmeyer and Karrie Shogren, the many layers of support at Springer, and the inspiring staff at the VIA Institute on Character and Columbia University's Spirituality Mind Body Institute.

We are grateful for many colleagues—practitioners and academics—who have joined us in this important work exploring, studying, applying, and championing character strengths and positive psychology for people with different kinds of disabilities/abilities. We cannot name everyone, but here are several who have influenced us, encouraged us, and displayed a supportive trust in us in this space: James Pawelski, Donna Mayerson, Kris Copeland, Matt Copeland, Tayyab Rashid, Helen Genova, Diane Weinbrandt, Jim Hudson, Neal Mayerson, Erik Carter, Jess Datu, Chathurika Kannangara, Cooper Woodard, Nirb Singh, David Giwerc, Brian Skotko, Wenche "Venka" Gazaille, Dan Collinson, Elizabeth Jennings, Eileen Henry, Erin Taylor, Jamie Emberson, Marjorie Aunos, Emre Umucu, Ariel Schwartz, Shin Matsuguma, Elizabeth Tuckwiller, Katie Curran, Susan Brownknight, Tim Vogt, Willie Jones, Joni Beasley, David Jespersen, Annette Stagge, Marissa Rowley, Cathy Parsons, Angus Skinner, Pam Saeks, Missy Skavlem, Cindy Gosh-Lee, Ron Margolis, Kathy Miller, and Danny Wedding.

It might seem obvious, but we would not be writing this book if it weren't for our clients, students, and family. Our clients inspired our hope, curiosity, and perspective with this work to discover what is possible and to see the bigger picture; our students inspired our love of learning to delve into the nuances of this work; and our families inspired our love, zest, and teamwork to infuse this work with passion and energy while working collaboratively.

Collectively, these aforementioned people pointed us to answer the question—what matters most for this book? Our answer: to bring the science and practice of what is best in humanity to those who are cast aside, seen in a limited or stereotypic view, and/or are vulnerable to greater persecution and suffering.

Contents

About the Authors

Ryan M. Niemiec is a leading international figure in character strengths that are found in all human beings. As a scientist, educator, and practitioner, Ryan is the Chief Science and Education Officer of the renown VIA Institute on Character, a nonprofit organization in Cincinnati, Ohio, that leads the global advancement of the science of character strengths. Ryan is an award-winning psychologist, annual instructor at the University of Pennsylvania, and author of 14 books and over 100 academic or peer-reviewed papers. His books include the bestselling *The Power of Character Strengths*, *Character Strengths Interventions*, and *Mindfulness and Character Strengths*. His research collaborations extend across the globe with more than 100 collaborators and approximately one million research participants. He is Fellow of the International Positive Psychology Association (IPPA), serves on their Council of Advisors, and is Co-Founder/President of their Spirituality/Meaning Division. In 2023, he was awarded the Raymond D. Fowler Service Award by IPPA. In the disability space, Ryan has co-authored several peer-reviewed papers including the flagship paper for the field that makes the case for the integration of character strengths for intellectual/developmental disability; has presented widely at local and national conferences; and has worked directly with hundreds of individuals spanning from intellectual/developmental disabilities, psychological disorders, and medical/physical disorders. His greatest teachers of character strengths are his children, one who has Down syndrome and two who have ADHD.

Dan Tomasulo is Academic Director at the Spirituality Mind Body Institute (SMBI), Teachers College, Columbia University. He holds a Ph.D. in Psychology, MFA in writing, and a Master of Applied Positive Psychology from the University of Pennsylvania. Formally a teaching fellow at Princeton, he is a Review Editor for *Frontiers in Psychology*, and honored by Teachers College, Columbia University, with their annual Teaching Award. He is the author of five books and co-author of American Psychological Association's first psychotherapy book for people with IDD. His award-winning memoir, *American Snake Pit*, unveils the hope, grit, and resilience of the inmates of America's most notorious asylum. Dan co-authored the

Diagnostic Manual—Intellectual Disability (DM-ID) section on identifying the criteria for Post-Traumatic Stress Disorder in people with IDD, and holds the NADD clinical certification to provide specialized treatment to these individuals. Dan is a fellow of the American Society for Group Psychotherapy/Psychodrama and honored as one of the top ten online influencers on depression. Twice awarded the Avant-Garde Clinical Intervention by the International Positive Psychology Association, he is the developer of Positive-Interactive Behavioral Therapy, a widely used form of group psychotherapy for people with IDD.

Part I
Foundations for Character Strengths and Disabilities

The chapters in Part I lay the foundation for the book. We target the value of strengths and strength-based approaches, and go into depth on one type of strength—character strengths.

Chapter 1 offers a wide lens on strengths, strengths-based approaches, and disability. It highlights the emergence of well-being approaches and enters a general discussion of why strengths are important for well-being. The reflections on the different kinds of strengths become critical in this chapter and for any discussion of disability, as the majority of focus is typically placed on strengths that are interests, skills, or resources of the person. It offers compelling scientific studies showing a focus on amplifying strengths is superior in many contexts to remediating deficits or weaknesses. The practical focus of the chapter tackles both strengths-based assessment and the shift to move from deficit to strengths.

Chapter 2 offers a foundation for the category of strengths known as character strengths. As character strengths are the central premise and discussion in every chapter of this book—from scientific and practical perspectives—a solid framework and review are needed. Therefore, core principles and scientific findings spanning multiple domains of life, well-being areas, and adversity areas are discussed, placing emphasis on the most researched and substantive system in the field known as the VIA classification of character strengths. A thorough conceptualization of a character strengths-based approach is outlined, followed by five character strengths interventions, case examples, and strategies around developing a character strengths practice.

Part I
Foundations for Character Strengths and Disorders

Chapter 1
Introduction to Disability and Strengths-Based Approaches

The Concepts

Every person on this planet—if they live long enough—will have a disability. There are no exceptions. Some people are born with a particular condition (e.g., cerebral palsy), for others it emerges over time (e.g., mental illnesses), for others it the result of a sudden accident (e.g., paraplegia), for others it is a medical condition that is unexpected (e.g., a heart attack) or progressive (e.g., many cases of diabetes), and for others it is a degenerative process in aging (e.g., Alzheimer's disease). Also consider the disabling impact for many people who had or have COVID-19, or a family member or friend who deeply suffered with it or passed away from it. When we see disability through such a wide lens, we realize no one escapes disability. It is part of the human condition.

Disabilities are on the rise. In the United States, disabilities are the largest minority group and increased by 25% from 1990 to 2000 (Disability Funders Network, 2022). Table 1.1 offers a few general statistics of disability by the numbers to help the reader understand the connection of disability to everyone. These statistics remind us of the realities of disability for each person, their family, and the collective society. These data also echo the insights of many scientists and practitioners who observe that disability is a natural part of the human experience (e.g., Carter, 2016).

In addition to the sheer numbers, there are unique physical and mental impacts on people with disability, depending on the type of disability. There is greater vulnerability to such problems for people from developing (i.e., majority world) countries, according to the World Report on Disability (Officer & Shakespeare, 2013).

Collectively, these statistics might engender a humble pause. Reflecting on the realities of temporary and long-term disabilities for ourselves and our loved ones, we understand we are interconnected with disability. We cannot separate ourselves

R. M. Niemiec, D. Tomasulo, *Character Strengths and Abilities Within Disabilities*, Positive Psychology and Disability Series,
https://doi.org/10.1007/978-3-031-36294-1_1

Table 1.1 The pervasiveness of disability[a]

Percentages	Reality
Over 1 billion (15%)	People in the world with a disability/health condition
26%	Adults in the United States have some type of disability
29%	People in the United States have at least one family member with a disability
40%	Adults over 65 in the United States have a disability
99%	Nearly every person knows someone with a disability
100%	All of us will have a disability if we live long enough

References: Line 1: World Health Organization (2021). Lines 2, 4: Centers for Disease Control (2018). Line 3: Disability Funders Network (2022). Lines 5, 6: These are logical conclusions we are drawing. They cast a wide net reflecting all the possible disabilities a person can experience

from it, nor can we escape it. This might create a few extra ounces of compassion, understanding, and empathy toward others.

Such understanding and empathy is at the heart of strengths-based approaches. It propels individuals to seek out the good, the positive, and the strong in all people and to connect with people in a way that is empowering, grounded, and hopeful.

Historically, disability has not been discussed or conceptualized in the context of strengths and capacities until fairly recently (Wehmeyer, 2013). Over recent decades, there have been a number of breakthroughs in the disability world such as the inclusion and anti-discrimination approaches advocated for in the Americans with Disabilities Act of 1990 and the movement toward approaches that are strengths-based with the Individuals with Disabilities Education Act (IDEA) and the requiring of individualized education plans (IEPs) in public schools in the United States. Another breakthrough came when the American Association on Intellectual and Developmental Disabilities (AAIDD) adopted a social-ecological approach to disability that described individuals' functioning as being not only about problems and weakness but strengths in different areas of functioning, and placed an emphasis on environmental considerations as well (Buntinx, 2013; Luckasson et al., 1992).

The various disabilities discuss in this book—intellectual/developmental, medical, mental, and physical disability—are largely discussed in categorical systems such as the *DSM-5* and the *ICD-11*. This illness ideology pervades psychology and social sciences, and especially clinical psychology (Maddux, 2009). These systems operate in all-or-none terms of the person having the condition or disorder or not. As Maddux (2009) explains, they operate under a number of faulty assumptions: categories are facts about the world, normal and abnormal can be distinguished, categories facilitate clinical judgment, and categories facilitate intervention. These dominant approaches in the lives of so many are both helpful (e.g., offering understanding, facilitating treatment options) and limiting (e.g., only describing part of the person; omitting what is going well). In contrast to categorical approaches, there are dimensional approaches to understanding symptoms and to understanding phenomena such as strengths. Dimensional approaches offer the frame of more or less and often make use of a continuum model where, in a particular context, a person displays more (or less) sadness and more (or less) curiosity; this approach opens the door for the myriad of possible situational scenarios and places an emphasis on the variation of individual differences.

The Science of Well-Being

There are a number of fields and disciplines that have conducted basic and applied research on well-being, strengths, positivity, and growth-oriented aspects of human functioning. Collectively these can be referred to as *positive psychology* or the *science of well-being*. Positive psychology is an umbrella term meant to be inclusive of the various positive areas within human beings, between human beings, and among institutions and societies where human beings work, play, and interact; therefore, positive psychology provides a substantial value-add focal point of study and practice because of the prevailing focus on what is wrong, disorder, disabled, or struggling (Seligman, 1999). Positive psychology does not replace or discount any other field or discipline, rather it integrates with and enhances what it is being integrated into. Positive psychology, especially character strengths, is not only about moving from what's wrong to what's strong, but is about using what's strong to deal with what's wrong or challenging or difficult. Said another way, a strength's focus engenders both a shift to strength and a shift to use strengths within and for suffering (Niemiec, 2023). Suffering can be a relationship conflict, a new medical diagnosis, a longstanding depression, a challenge in understanding another's speech, the experience of trauma, or a seemingly infinite array of possible challenges, hardships, disorders, and stressors.

Positive psychology and well-being approaches offer scientific measurement and interventions in well-being to the area or field of focus, such as social work, counseling, public policy, school inclusiveness, transition/employment opportunities, or any other area studying or supporting people with a disability.

One of the original core areas in the field of positive psychology—and often referred to as the "backbone of positive psychology"—is the study of character traits, or character strengths (Seligman, 1999). Character strengths are integrated into each of the subsequent chapters that follow Chap. 2, which is the other foundational chapter. In this chapter, however, we will keep our focus more broad to "strengths" in general, yet draw some distinctions therein.

Why Strengths?

Our brain is wired for what is wrong, seeing flaws/problems/dangers (i.e., fight or flight system) in our environment. Research consistently shows that bad is stronger and more powerful than the good, in terms of our health, parenting, emotions, thinking, habits, and a host of other psychological and social phenomena (Baumeister et al., 2001). Other research has similarly focused on the pervasiveness of negativity observing findings that negativity is stronger than the positive, it grows faster than the positive, it dominates the positive, and is more varied and complex than the positive (Rozin & Royzman, 2001). These extensive findings form an imbalance priming us to focus on problems, suffering, and difficulties and omit what is going well, is strong, or is positive in life. Additional research shows that people perceive their weaknesses as more malleable than their strengths and, in turn, tend to believe they will improve or correct their weaknesses as opposed to their strengths (Steimer & Mata, 2016). This research points to the natural inclination for people to prioritize weaknesses and flaws.

This research points to the critical need for strengths and the impact it can have in counterbalancing our natural inclinations and biases.

To further the argument for the importance of strengths, we turn to studies pointing to problematically high percentages of disengagement and strength blindness, alongside studies that show the role of strengths for flourishing. See Table 1.2 for data pointing to the stark distinction.

Next, we make some important distinctions by taking a closer look at the different kinds of strengths that human beings have. These represent different ways of working with and thinking about strengths.

There Are Many Kinds of Strengths

The term "strengths" has become a commonplace, go-to term in the disability field. When a person, group, or organization is using the term strengths without specifying the "type" of strength they are focusing on, we label these as *generic strengths*. In other words, the practitioner, educator, or researcher is attempting to help another

Table 1.2 Suffering, flourishing, and strengths, by the numbers

	Finding	Citation
Suffering	2/3 of people do not have a meaningful awareness of their strengths (UK)	Linley (2008)
	80% of people are not flourishing (United States)	Keyes (2003)
	87% of people are not engaged in their work (global)	Crabtree (2013)
Flourishing	High strengths awareness = 9× more likely to be flourishing than low strengths awareness (New Zealand)	Hone et al. (2015)
	High strengths use = 18× more likely to be flourishing than low strengths use (New Zealand)	Hone et al. (2015)
	Workers using 4 or more top strengths are significantly more likely to have positive work experiences and work-as-a-calling (Europe)	Harzer and Ruch (2015)
	Strengths training directly increases work engagement, personal resources, and strengths use (Europe)	Bakker and van Wingerden (2020)

Note: In this table, "high" means highest quartile and "low" means lowest quartile person with something positive, good, or growth-oriented that is often (but not always) within the person. But, one thing has become clear in the world of strengths: There are many categories or types of strengths. The generality—and often vagueness—of generic strengths can be quickly differentiated from approaches that clarify the specific type of strengths of a person. This means to label and be aware of the type of strength being focused on. For this discussion, we draw upon the following categories from Niemiec (2018): talents (abilities or intelligences), skills (competencies), interests (passions), values, resources, and character strengths.

There are strengths of *talent or ability* that encompass what we do naturally well. A good example of this is Howard Gardner's (1983) multiple intelligences which include being strong with intelligences such as spatial reasoning, mathematical/logical ability, interpersonal relating, and musical intelligence, to name a few. Although talents are substantially biologically loaded, they require extensive practice to bring them to highest fruition, with some researchers estimating about 10 years containing 10,000 h of practice (Ericsson & Ward, 2007). The loss of such talents can be devastating if one considers the college football player with tremendous bodily/kinesthetic talent who sustains a spinal cord injury rendering them unable to play football professionally. That same football player, tapping into a strengths mindset, might decide to utilize their bodily/kinesthetic talent in a different form by joining one of the many international wheelchair rugby teams that play competitively. Individuals with autism-spectrum disorder are frequently stereotyped as having a special "talent" such as memorizing large amounts of information, having unusual and stunning abilities with numbers, trivia, maps, or obscure information, and it has been estimated that about 10% of people with autism have such savant qualities (Teffert, 2009).

Another type of strength is *skills*, also referred to as competencies that one develops. Skills develop through learning and practice and are a means to an end, such as learning communication skills in order to get a job or learning computer programming skills in order to get a promotion. When a person has a disability, there are usually a number of skills that are important for them to adapt and grow. A person with depression will need to learn the skill of behavioral activation (Mazzucchelli et al., 2010) whether that be through walking, exercising, or engaging in pleasurable activities. A person with paraplegia will need to learn the skill of navigating their wheelchair and building their upper body strength therein, and executive functioning skills involving planning as they navigate areas of their community that may or may not be accessible.

The strength category of *interests* reflects passions in life. Each person has leisure time and how they choose to spend it will often reflect their areas of interest. Perhaps they spend their free time reading, playing video games, engaging in art or music, volunteering at a nature group, or talking with friends. Whatever a person's disability, there is a way to tap into their interests. For example, a person who has some confines of mobility who also has a passion for wildlife can watch documentaries of wildlife, be supported with a friend by engaging in nature, having discussions with friends or community members about local wildlife, and/or looking into ways they can advocate for wildlife protection (through writing, promotion of positive activities, or active participation in groups).

We define the strength category referred to as *resources* as those supports (e.g., devices, people, networks) that are external to us (the other categories are internal). There are a myriad of examples of general resources such as living in a safe neighborhood, and having caring family members, friends, and helping professionals. Other resources serve as tools such as wheelchairs, safety harnesses on buses, diabetes test kits, electronic communication devices, Braille transcription services, and so on. Any tool or support that helps an individual to live their daily life at home, work, social, and/or in relationships more fully or easily or helps them engage more directly in the community could be considered a resource. Self-determination approaches weigh heavily on helping individuals tap into their external resources, among other strengths categories (Shogren, 2013; Wehmeyer, 2005). The importance of the individual's culture is another strength resource to be discussed/encouraged—and is both an internal asset and external. We discuss it here under resources as many cultural elements are external such as the cultural elements of community, food/drink, traditions/rituals, and stories; some internal elements of culture include cultural values, expression of language, certain cultural skills, and (again) stories. An individual's creativity, zest, and honesty/authenticity can allow their cultural beliefs, artistic expression, culinary expression, and other rituals to shine in the family and community.

Values can be viewed as a type of strength and are probably the most vague and amorphous of all the categories. One can "value" any of the types of strengths discussed (e.g., one might value the strength of bravery, having the resource of many friends, one's own communication skills, interest in bowling, or guitar-playing ability). As values refer to our internal cognitive and emotional care and energy toward what matters to us, values do not refer to our actual behaviors, commitments, goals, or actions that we take. Many schools of thought place emphasis on values (e.g., acceptance and commitment therapy) and it is clear that to make the most of values, one must explicitly note that the intention is "values in action" or "commitment to one's values," as values-alone is not enough.

While conceptually there appears to be plenty of distinctiveness between each category, there have not been research studies conducted on all the categories together to determine any degree of overlap, unique correlates, expressions, and consequences of each. Therefore, at this time in the psychological science, we are left to rely on conceptual distinctions. The science of strengths will deepen by understanding and examining these categories more closely.

In many disability spaces, these aforementioned categories are the most common areas of strength that are explored and intervened upon. That said, we posit that the most important type of strength for practitioners, educators, researchers, parents, advocates, leaders, and policy makers to focus on is strengths of character. Yet, it is the category least focused on in education and practice in the disability fields, and thereby is one of the causative factors for assembling this book. Chapter 2 will lay the foundation for the science and practice of character strengths and Chaps. 3, 4, 5, 6, 7, 8, 9, and 10 will focus on the integration of character strengths into the area of disability or topic area being discussed. For this chapter, we largely stay with "strengths" as meaning "generic strengths."

The Science

Strengths or Deficits?

Consider two groups: One group is asked to focus on their weaknesses or deficits and to try to improve them. The other group is asked to focus on their strengths and to try to improve them. Which approach do you think is more common in helping people with disabilities? Which approach might lead to better outcomes? Researchers are beginning to compare these two groups of amplifying strengths and remediating/correcting deficits in head-to-head groups in randomized studies. The results will surprise some readers. Across the studies, it is the amplifying strengths/positives approach that is emerging with higher benefit. Here are seven studies that have tested this comparison.

- In outpatient treatment centers, greater benefits for anxiety, stress, depression, suicidal ideation, and positive affect were found for the positive affect treatment group in comparison with the negative affect treatment group (Craske et al., 2019).
- A clinical study focusing on individuals diagnosed with major depressive disorder had therapists focus on building strengths or remediating deficits in the cognitive-behavioral treatment context. The group randomly assigned to building strengths led to better outcomes and quicker recovery than the group focused on deficit-reduction (Cheavens et al., 2012).
- Across five studies, individuals learned more from success than from failure, even when incentives were provided for learning (Eskreis-Winkler & Fishbach, 2019).
- Among students preparing for exams, the prevention of negative emotions and distress prior to exams and optimism about the future were significant for only the strengths group (Dolev-Amit et al., 2020).
- Among graduate students, focusing on strengths led to greater increases in personal growth in the short-term (but not the long-term) while focuses on correcting deficits had no impact on personal growth. A second study found larger benefits in personal growth than deficit correction after 3 months (Meyers et al., 2015).
- Across two studies, individuals focused on professional development engaged in strategies to develop their relative strengths or to improve their perceived weaknesses. The strengths group consistently showed higher levels of competence, intrinsic motivation, and effort intentions compared with the group focusing on weaknesses (Hiemstra & Van Yperen, 2015).
- In the work context, perceived organizational support for strengths use connected strongly with self-ratings and manager-ratings of job performance, while perceived organizational support for deficit correction was unrelated to job performance (van Woerkom et al., 2016).

Some of these studies included people with disabilities (e.g., depression), some did not. Nevertheless, they collectively make the scientific finding that to focus only on what is wrong is to miss an important part of the equation. Moreover, deficits may actually be less important than strengths. These studies do not offer a foregone conclusion of preferring strengths over deficits nor do they suggest this is the optimal approach in all situations. Rather, they encourage new thinking and balanced approaches for researchers, practitioners, and systems striving to boost well-being while supporting suffering.

Strengths-Based Approaches Across Disciplines

While the conducting of scientific experiences on strengths is relatively new, there has been plenty of scholarly discussion preceding these studies. Theorizing on strengths and linking them with quality practice has been discussed for more than two decades and spans many fields.

In the social work field, Dennis Saleebey (1996) was an early pioneer of strengths orientations, theorizing, and application into social work. His focus also included strengths-based case management for people with severe mental illness (Saleebey, 1992). In the psychotherapy world, the pioneering work of Carl Rogers brought a focus to person-centered work and a focus on the humanness of people (Rogers, 1961). More recently, it has been Tayyab Rashid who has championed the weaving of character strengths into psychotherapy, emphasizing a counterbalance to what's wrong by infusing a focus on both deficits and strengths (Rashid & Seligman, 2019).

Strengths-based approaches are varied and have been studied and applied in leadership (Welch et al., 2014), with high-risk youth (Arnold et al., 2007), in workplace coaching (Peláez et al., 2020), in nursing (Gottlieb & Gottlieb, 2017), in counseling (Smith, 2006), in supervision (Lietz & Julien-Chinn, 2017), in organizational work (Cooperrider & Whitney, 2005), in mindfulness (Niemiec, 2014), in project management (Pearce, 2018), in executive coaching (Foster & Auerbach, 2015), and in education (Linkins et al., 2015). Note that this is not an exhaustive list nor is there one pathway, model, or theoretical orientation for describing a strengths-based approach. However, unifying approaches have been theorized and proposed (see Niemiec & Pearce, 2021), which will be discussed in subsequent chapters.

In the disability field, a strengths-based approach focuses on the person, the human being, first, and arguably that means to see who they are—their character strengths, as prioritized as the focal point in Niemiec et al. (2017). Strengths-based approaches focus on what the person can do instead of giving only attention to what they cannot do, examining what is strong instead of limiting attention to what is wrong, and prioritizing growth, the positive, and empowerment. Self-determination approaches have been a leading, strength-focused approach in the disability field. Self-determination approaches are strengths-based approaches in the disability field that create alignment between the person's capacities and their environment (Wehmeyer, 2020). Such approaches involve purposeful, intentional actions in which the individual is the causal agent to make things happen in their lives that helps them improve or maintain their well-being or quality of life (Wehmeyer, 2005). In other words, the individual is the author of their life and has control to aspire toward their goals (Wehmeyer & Little, 2013). There are a variety of strength-skills individuals can develop to make good choices, manage themselves and self-advocate, and reach their goals (Shogren, 2013).

Stigma and Strengths

Stigma of people with disabilities is prevalent. Perhaps no disability group is exempt from the immediate or persisting negative judgments by others and the often negative personal attributions and imposed limitations by others. Mental health stigma has been examined and found that social intelligence and kindness were associated with less stigma, while those with judgment/critical thinking were less likely to hold those with disorders personally responsible for acquiring the condition (Vertilo & Gibson, 2014).

Datu and Niemiec (2023) investigated over 21,000 individuals in the general public and their personal contact with people with different kinds of disabilities, their character strengths, and their stigmatization levels of people in four disability categories—autism, intellectual/developmental disability, mental illness, and physical disability. Several patterns emerged including the character of strengths of kindness, fairness, social intelligence, and love of learning being associated most strongly with less stigma; there were also patterns of consistently strong associations with less stigma across disabilities and the strengths of leadership, bravery, love, appreciation of beauty, curiosity, and humor. Perseverance, self-regulation, and spirituality were generally associated with higher levels of stigma. These general findings reflect the value of a mindset and approach toward people that is inclusive (fairness), involves warmth, caring, empathy, humanity, and other-orientedness (love, kindness, and social intelligence), playfulness and lightheartedness (humor), a seeing of the good in little things (appreciation of beauty), a desire to explore and learn about others (love of learning and curiosity), and a willingness to guide others and move out of one's comfort zone (leadership and bravery). On the other hand, strengths that might be more closely associated with a self-focus (e.g., perseverance, self-regulation) or looking beyond the person (e.g., spirituality) might be more likely to facilitate patterns of greater stigmatization. These are correlational findings and therefore might serve as signposts toward areas warranting further investigation, potential insight, and eventual interventions, and are not conclusions about any individual's strength patterns and whether they will or will not stigmatize others, nor do they reflect the complex interplay these character strengths unfold systemically and synergistically within an individual.

The Practice

If you are an educator, practitioner, or person who supports one or many people with a disability, consider this simple question: Are you strengths-based?

We have found in querying thousands of practitioners in workshops across the globe and across spheres of application (e.g., consultants and coaches in the workplace, teachers and professors in education, and counselors, social workers, and psychologists in clinics and hospitals) that the vast majority raise a hand signifying a "yes." They endorse themselves as a strengths-based practitioner or as having a strengths-based practice. Who wants to proclaim they are not "strengths-based"? The implication is that one is otherwise a "deficit-based practitioner." And, there are a wide range of good things about human beings and a wide range of ways to approach that goodness, hence there are plenty of "strengths" areas to explore. We give attention to the characteristics of a strengths-based approach and a strengths-based practitioner in Chap. 2. Here, we turn to approaches in strengths-based assessment.

In strengths-based assessment, there is an emphasis on balance in the exploration, namely, around the integration of strengths with weaknesses. This has been articulated in consulting (Berg, 2009) and psychotherapy (Rashid & Ostermann, 2009) contexts. Berg argues for an approach that focuses on strengths/assets in the client and in the environment, as well as weaknesses in the client and in the environment. The widening to strengths adds a necessary complexity to understanding the individual while the addition of the environment offers the opportunity for the practitioner to better understand the source of the individual's strengths and problems (Wright & Lopez, 2009).

Buntinx (2013) expands some of these concepts to the disability sphere and suggests a functional approach to strengths. This four-phase approach includes the following:

1. Assessment of the individual's strengths and weaknesses in functioning. This involves healthy and strong functioning areas and positive potentials as well as activity limitations, medical/health conditions, and other impairments.
2. Assessment of the individual's ambitions, desires, and needs.
3. Individualized support planning that focuses on the individual's goals, activities to reach those goals, and supports and resources to help get them there.
4. Review of past/present support efforts in terms of the individual's quality of life, with the intention of improving supports.

Another area of strengths-based assessment to explore is to consider each of the strength categories within the person and how they fare on each. Therefore, we shift back to our earlier discussion on the types of strengths and consider strengths-based assessment questions for each area, along with examples. See Table 1.3. Note that some assessment questions would need to be adjusted based on the type of disability the individual is experiencing.

Table 1.3 Assessing the different kinds of strengths

Strength area	Description	Assessment questions	Comments	Examples
Talents/ abilities	Hard-wired, innate capacities	What are you good at? What comes most natural to you? What do others say you are really good at?	Although probably not as malleable as the other categories, these can be tapped into and grown over time with practice	Bodily/kinesthetic, verbal, musical, interpersonal, intrapersonal, spatial reasoning, mathematical/logical reasoning
Skills/ competencies	Proficiencies acquired as a means to an end	What skills have you developed for your job? What daily tasks have you learned to do well? What helps you to best communicate with people?	These are important for work, school, and self-care management and growth	Personal (anger management and communication skills); job-related (typing skills, public speaking skills); school-related (attentiveness skills; study practice skills); social (initiation skills, listening skills, empathy skills)
Interests/ passions	Activities and leisure areas that the person feels compelled to do	What do you like to do in your free time? What are you most excited to do at home? What is most fun for you to do?	These are particularly relatable for each individual and thereby draws interest and excitement to discuss	Art, blogging, collecting, exercising/ walking, games, languages, photography, social media, sports, travel, writing, volunteering, yoga
Resources	External supports to help, guide, or sustain a person at work, school, community, home	Who supports you at home? Who supports you in community or at work? What supports are in place to help you do your job better or attend classes more smoothly?	These are myriad and help to better align the person with the environment, especially when the environment cannot or will not change	Family, neighbors/ community, friends, medical staff, psychology staff, disability support team, volunteer group, support groups, spiritual/religious community, safety of living environment, access to resources in community, transportation, accessibility equipment (e.g., wheelchair, crutches)

(continued)

Table 1.3 (continued)

Strength area	Description	Assessment questions	Comments	Examples
Values	Aspects of life that are instinctively motivating and the person holds as dear to them	What do you hold as important or dear to you? What drives you to take action in your life?	Values live in our thinking and feeling (they do not necessarily reflect action). It is a general term that overlaps with other categories—one can value one's character strengths, resources, etc.	Hard work, freedom, family, simplicity, integrity, friendship, justice, tradition, understanding, wealth, commitment, community, environment, ethics, service, spirituality, self-respect, inclusion, independence (to name a few)
Character	Positive personality qualities that reflect core identity, produce positive outcomes, and contribute to the greater good	What is best about who you are? In what ways are you a good person? What are the qualities that help you to thrive? To be resilient? What is an example of when you did something good for others?	Character lives in our thinking, feeling, volition/ willing, and behavior. This category is the fuel for all the other categories	Appreciating beauty, bravery, creativity, curiosity, fairness, forgiveness, gratitude, honesty, humor, humility, hope, judgment, kindness, love, love of learning, leadership, perseverance, perspective, prudence, self-regulation, social intelligence, spirituality, teamwork, zest

The category of character is viewed as the driving force for each of the other categories (Niemiec, 2018). Character strengths help the other categories to operate. For example, if someone has a musical intelligence/talent for playing the piano, they need to regularly and deeply use their character strengths of self-regulation (discipline), prudence (planning out their practice periods amidst other activities), perseverance (keeping up the practice), hope (seeing the future in which they are successfully playing piano), creativity (keeping the practice fresh and fun), zest (maintaining a positive energy in practice), and other character strengths. Without character strengths, the talent would surely fizzle. The same is true for the other categories of strength, such as the person's character strength of love of learning to develop new skills, curiosity to pursue their interests, and social intelligence to tap into their resources.

Moving from Deficit to Strength

Building from the research discussed in this chapter, it is clear that turning to strengths is an important and often forgotten element. Sometimes the focus on strengths is a complement to a focus on what is wrong and sometimes it is a reframing or shift from what is wrong.

The following are personal stories relating to the practical importance and ramifications of shifting the focus to strengths. They emphasize both positive reappraisal (e.g., Garland et al., 2011) and a focus on the individual themselves, which is among the main recommendations in the World Report on Disability offered to the World Health Organization (Officer & Shakespeare, 2013).

One of my (RMN) sons has Down syndrome. Compared to the typically developing child, he was delayed in holding himself up, sitting, crawling, standing, and walking. In fact, his delay in movement led him to completely skip the crawling phase when he was young. He would only scoot across the floor (moving on his butt with his legs and hands). During that phase several years ago, I was picking him up from daycare and he was the last child in the room. One day, I stood and observed him playing with some blocks and began chatting with his daycare teacher. Soon, he recognized the sound of my voice, turned around, and began to scoot over to me. I made an offhanded comment to the teacher that I wished he was walking like his peers. Without hesitation, the teacher exclaimed, "Well, his scooting gets the job done! He gets wherever he wants to go. If other kids are playing on the other side of the room, he gets there." While I had previously understood that point, her comment hit me in a more direct and meaningful way. She was handing me a positive reframe that reflected a reality that had been right under my nose or had been in a faded, preconscious part of my mind. I had not been viewing the reality that his scooting was a positive behavior. It was meeting his needs and giving him a feeling of accomplishment. It was indeed a great strength.

This conversation led me to converse more with the teacher and we came to the point of mutually observing that my son was actually very fast at scooting. "Sometimes he gets to places quicker than his peers can walk there!" she exclaimed. "And," she joked, "he doesn't fall." This teacher's observation helped me further this growing insight with positive reappraisal. I paid a lot more attention to his scooting, with a lens of joy, curiosity, and gratitude. I began to appreciate it each time he scooted, as it was something positive and indeed, he was a very fast scooter! Of course, I wanted to see him walking but I reminded myself that that was more my aspiration than his; he was doing just fine as he was. He was not only getting his needs met but he was meeting his needs himself and he seemed to feel empowered in doing so. As the parent, I strove to strengthen my mind toward a positive default in my observations and interactions with my son, leaning me toward becoming a more strengths-based parent.

I (DT) was embarrassed by my reactions as a teenager to people with emotional disabilities. I could feel an initial reaction, a type of repugnance that pushed me back—somehow shut me down. I became quieter, avoiding, ignoring, or turning away from the individual. I did not understand this reaction, but it troubled me. What was I so afraid of? What jammed my normal way of being? While I first noticed this with people whose emotions seemed off, they yelled too loud, or were social awkward, I found this type of reaction also happened with people with physical disabilities. It troubled me that I would have this response—an embarrassment of sorts. Nothing else in my adolescent experiences caused this type of effect.

There was a man in my hometown, Richie, who was intellectually disabled and mentally ill. He was also slightly disfigured, with a very large nose, and walked with unusual speed. He was made fun of by students, shunned by parents, and hidden from children. Yet, Richie was a fan of all the high school sports teams. He always seemed unfettered by the antics of others, and he said hello and waved to you if there was eye contact. His constant presence at the high school football, basketball, wrestling, and baseball events always seemed to bring mocking ridicule, unflattering mimicking, and derogatory statements: Go home idiot! "Looser!" and the cruel mimicry of teenagers were constant taunts. On occasion there would be the lone parent or teacher or coach who would yell; "knock it off," but it never really got better. Richie would show up, yell for his team: "Come on, you, can do it, you can do it!" He also had a slight lisp, and would occasionally stutter, which made even his cheering something that caused an offensive remark or reaction. When I saw Richie at these events I wondered why he would be there. Why would someone put themselves into such a vulnerable and exposed circumstance? I felt bad for him, but also wished he would not make himself a target. Why not stay home? Or be quiet? Or sit somewhere else, but the middle of the bleachers? In other words: Why don't you make *my* life easier by not being *you*.

As Richie made his presence known people would either shut down like me, or act out like those mocking him. His presence caused people to react. Even the parents and teachers and coaches trying to keep the peace were affected. People were not neutral around him. What I did not notice was any sweetness toward him. No one said hello, no one smiled, no one shook his hand. I noticed people's reactions, but I also seemed shut down—I never did anything sweet, or kind toward him either.

Richie was ubiquitous. It did not matter if we were dropping my sister off for dance lessons, or getting Friday night pizza, or food shopping. Richie was there, and he always seemed to be in a good mood, and always walking off in a hurry. On occasion he would try to start a conversation with a teenage girl—but this almost always ended by the young girl turning away without saying anything, or after a polite, but curt, hello. A few of these encounters ended with the girls saying awful things to him about his appearance or speech, but never once did I see a mean or negative reaction from him. In fact, the only thing I ever heard Richie reply to anything ever said to him was: "That's okay, that's okay." There wasn't a mean bone in his body.

Toward the end of high school I took a job at an ice cream parlor in town and in fairly short order became the manager—helping to make the ice cream, opening up, closing up, and cleaning up. I took some pride in managing it and the owner and I got along very well. Over time he gave me more responsibilities and pay—and of course there was the added bonus that I could have a helping of anything I wanted at the end of my shift. My friends and fellow students would come in. It was a perfect way to make some money, be around my friends, and eat some terrific ice cream.

One day Richie came in and ordered a rum raisin ice cream cone. I served it up for him and while I was holding the cone out for him to take, he began the excruciating process of counting out the 30 cents in pennies, nickels, and dimes. He was short by three cents and I told him not to worry about it. A customer saw our exchange and told Richie to put his money away and that the cone was a treat from him. This was the first act of kindness I had seen happen to Richie. As the man handed me the money Richie froze, not knowing what to say or do—genuinely shocked. While I held out the cone Richie gathered up his change on the counter and stuffed it back in his pocket. His moistened eyes darted back and forth between the customer and me. He took the cone from my hand and started vigorously shaking his head—a type of humbled, animated thank you to both of us. In what seemed like one synchronized move he started eating the ice cream, quickly walked toward the door, and muttered: "That's okay, that's okay." Richie had no idea how to receive kindness.

Richie then showed up every day. It was as though kindness and good fortune were now linked to the ice cream parlor and he would be there soon after I opened, buy a rum raisin ice cream, and stay long after he was done. After a while the owner realized this, thought it was bad for business, and told me I had to tell Richie he could not stay once he finished his ice cream. I did this, and explained the seats were for people eating their ice cream and once done he would have to go so someone else could sit. Richie understood, but when he left he stayed right outside the door. The owner was not happy about this new turn of events and told me he was going to get the police involved. For several days we discussed alternate means to handle the situation, and along the way I recommended hiring Richie to help clean up. This way he could be connected to the ice cream parlor, I would have him help me in the evenings, and we could tell him part of the deal is not to hang around during the day. The owner rejected this idea out of hand and it was clear the police would soon be involved.

Then the unimaginable happened. Out of the blue the owner's wife, only 38 years old, died of a brain aneurism and we closed the store for a week. Everyone in town knew her and the funeral parlor was packed every night. On the last night Richie was in the back holding rosaries. When the owner thanked him for coming Richie's eyes darted around. "That's okay, that's okay," was, again, all he could say.

After that the owner hired Richie to help me clean up the nights I closed the shop. He was a hard worker and it cut the time it usually took me in half. We fell into a routine of cleaning the ice cream machine, wiping the soda fountain down, cleaning all the dishes, then putting the chairs on top of the tables and mopping the floor. Richie stayed away during the day—yet faithfully showed up at night. As the floor was drying we would sit and eat a well-deserved ice cream cone. I would usually have chocolate chip, and Richie loyally chose his rum raisin.

Then one day Richie did not show: Then not again—and again. There were rumors about what happened: He had gotten hit by a car walking at night; he was hospitalized in an institution; he ran away. I always wondered what happened to him. Although I tried finding out, I never saw him again and soon left the ice cream parlor for college and then graduate school.

So, I suppose, my career and calling and my invitation by Ryan to join him in writing this book is, in many ways, inspired by Richie. He was the first person I had direct connection with who struggled with intellectual and psychiatric disabilities. His innocence and enthusiasm for life, his ignorance and willingness to learn, and his desire for relationship opened my eyes and heart to people I had closed myself off to. What I learned from him and from the people I have worked with is that in spite of enormous intellectual and psychiatric disabilities these individuals are not very different from you and me. They crave love, need affection, compassion, and kindness, get hurt when they feel left out, are in need of guidance, want meaningful relationships, get angry when they are betrayed or cannot have their needs met, and are generally as confused and uncertain about their course in life as the rest of us.

As a psychologist learning what unites us as human beings and gives us the best tools for hope has been a quest since my first psychology course. When I first learned the power and elegance behind character strengths it was the first time I felt psychology had hit upon a universal language for cultivating the best inside us. I only wish they had been around when I knew Richie.[1]

Future Directions

Looking back a few decades—or even one decade—it is exciting to see how far strengths and strengths-based approaches have come. It is equally exciting to imagine the "long way to go" and the future possibilities in empowering all helpers to develop and maximize a strengths-based approach to help others build well-being and relationships and also to help them manage conflict, struggles, and problems.

An immediate area of growth for strengths psychology is in the integration of assessment—and ultimately interventions for—the various kinds of strengths within people of all abilities. A first step is for practitioners and systems to become clearer on what type of strength is being focused upon; any of the strength categories can be labeled, explored, and intervened upon. Related to this is the importance of differentiating how each type of strength develops over time, is malleable to change, and offers different consequences for use. A natural question alongside these areas of future investigation is how do the strengths categories come together? Might the combination of, for example, character strengths, talents, and interests align into what might be a powerful, internal strengths synergy? Further, how might positive interventions play a role in not only intervening upon each of these areas but also upon one strength area to then accentuate and influence the other strengths areas.

[1] A version of the above section appears in *American Snake Pit, Hope Grit and Resilience in the Wake of Willowbrook.*

Key Takeaways

- Disability is pervasive—most human beings themselves or their families/ friends have been impacted by a disability, and all people will be impacted if they live long enough.
- Human beings are wired to focus on what is wrong and to take on a negativity or deficit-based mindset. A focus on strengths provides an important realistic and honest counterbalance.
- Human beings have many different kinds of strengths—talents/abilities, skills/competencies, interests/passions, resources/supports, values, and character strengths. Character strengths are viewed as the foundation to enable, enrich, and/or drive the other strength areas.
- Across at least seven studies in which a focus on strengths was compared to a focus on weaknesses/deficits, the strengths group fared better on the outcomes in every study.
- Regardless of the type of strength being focused on, there are several approaches to strengths-based assessment that are useful, such as functional approaches and approaches that balance strengths/weakness in oneself and in one's environment.
- Practitioners can begin to shift their focus from deficit to strengths by taking a strengths-based mindset and using positive reappraisal.

References

Arnold, E. M., Walsh, A. K., Oldham, M. S., & Rapp, C. A. (2007). Strengths-based case management: Implementation with high-risk youth. *Families in Society, 88*(1), 86–94. https://doi.org/10.1606/1044-3894.3595

Bakker, A. B., & van Wingerden, J. (2020). Do personal resources and strengths use increase work engagement? The effects of a training intervention. *Journal of Occupational Health Psychology*. https://doi.org/10.1037/ocp0000266

Baumeister, R. F., Bratslavsky, E., Finkenaeuer, C., & Vohs, K. D. (2001). Bad is stronger than good. *Review of General Psychology, 5*(4), 323–370. https://doi.org/10.1037/1089-2680.5.4.323

Berg, C. J. (2009). A comprehensive framework for conducting client assessments: Highlighting strengths, environmental factors and hope. *Journal of Practical Consulting, 3*(2), 9–13.

Buntinx, W. H. E. (2013). Understanding disability: A strengths-based approach. In M. L. Wehmeyer (Ed.), *The Oxford handbook of positive psychology and disability* (pp. 7–18). Oxford University Press.

Carter, E. W. (2016). A place of belonging: Research at the intersection of faith and disability. *Review and Expositor, 113*(2), 167–180.

Centers for Disease Control and Prevention. (2018). *Disability and health data system (DHDS)*. Available from: http://dhds.cdc.gov. Accessed on 23 Sept 2022.

Cheavens, J. S., Strunk, D. R., Lazarus, S. A., & Goldstein, L. A. (2012). The compensation and capitalization models: A test of two approaches to individualizing the treatment of depression. *Behaviour Research and Therapy, 50*, 699–706.

Cooperrider, D., & Whitney, D. (2005). *Appreciative inquiry: A positive revolution in change*. Berrett-Koehler.

Crabtree, S. (2013). *Worldwide, 13% of employees are engaged at work*. Gallup. Found at: https://news.gallup.com/poll/165269/worldwide-employees-engaged-work.aspx

Craske, M. G., Meuret, A. E., Ritz, T., Treanor, M., Dour, H., & Rosenfield, D. (2019). Positive affect treatment for depression and anxiety: A randomized clinical trial for a core feature of anhedonia. *Journal of Consulting and Clinical Psychology, 87*(5), 457–471. https://doi.org/10.1037/ccp0000396

Datu, J., & Niemiec, R. M. (2023). *Disability: Character strengths, stigma, and acceptance across different disabilities*. Data from 21,800 people, collected on the VIA Institute on Character website.

Disability Funders Network. (2022). *Disability stats and facts*. Available at https://www.disabilityfunders.org/disability-stats-and-facts. Accessed on 23 Sept 2022.

Dolev-Amit, T., Rubin, A., & Zilcha-Mano, S. (2020). Is awareness of strengths intervention sufficient to cultivate wellbeing and other positive outcomes? *Journal of Happiness Studies*. https://doi.org/10.1007/s10902-020-00245-5

Ericsson, K. A., & Ward, P. (2007). Capturing the naturally occurring superior performance of experts in the laboratory: Toward a science of expert and exceptional performance. *Current Directions in Psychological Science, 16*(6), 346–350. https://doi.org/10.1111/j.1467-8721.2007.00533.x

Eskreis-Winkler, L., & Fishbach, A. (2019). Not learning from failure—The greatest failure of all. *Psychological Science, 30*, 1733. https://doi.org/10.1177/0956797619881133

Foster, S. L., & Auerbach, J. E. (2015). Positive psychology in coaching: Applying science to executive and personal coaching. Executive College Press.

Gardner, H. (1983). *Frames of mind: The theory of multiple intelligences*. Basic Books.

Garland, E. L., Gaylord, S. A., & Fredrickson, B. L. (2011). Positive reappraisal mediates the stress-reductive effects of mindfulness: An upward spiral process. *Mindfulness, 2*(1), 59–67. https://doi.org/10.1007/s12671-011-0043-8

Gottlieb, L. N., & Gottlieb, B. (2017). Strengths-based nursing: A process for implementing a philosophy into practice. *Journal of Family Nursing, 23*(3), 319–340. https://doi.org/10.1177/1074840717717731

Harzer, C., & Ruch, W. (2015). The relationships of character strengths with coping, work-related stress, and job satisfaction. Frontiers in Psychology, 6. https://doi.org/10.3389/fpsyg.2015.00165

Hiemstra, D., & Van Yperen, N. W. (2015). The effects of strength-based versus deficit-based self-regulated learning strategies on students' effort intentions. *Motivation and Emotion, 39*, 656–668. https://doi.org/10.1007/s11031-015-9488-8

Hone, L. C., Jarden, A., Duncan, S., & Schofield, G. M. (2015). Flourishing in New Zealand workers: Associations with lifestyle behaviors, physical health, psychosocial, and work-related indicators. *Journal of Occupational and Environmental Medicine, 57*(9), 973–983. https://doi.org/10.1097/JOM.0000000000000508

Keyes, C. L. M. (2003). Complete mental health: An agenda for the 21st century. In C. L. M. Keyes & J. Haidt (Eds.), *Flourishing: Positive psychology and the life well-lived* (pp. 293–312). American Psychological Association.

Lietz, C. A., & Julien-Chinn, F. J. (2017). Do the components of strengths-based supervision enhance child welfare workers' satisfaction with supervision? *Families in Society, 98*(2), 146–155. https://doi.org/10.1606/1044-3894.2017.98.20

Linkins, M., Niemiec, R. M., Gillham, J., & Mayerson, D. (2015). Through the strengths lens: A framework for educating the heart. *Journal of Positive Psychology, 10*(1), 64–68. https://doi.org/10.1080/17439760.2014.888581

Linley, A. (2008). *Average to A+: Realising strengths in yourself and others*. CAPP Press.

Luckasson, R., Coulter, D. L., Polloway, E. A., Reiss, S., Schalock, R. L., Snell, M. E., et al. (1992). *Mental retardation: Definition, classification, and systems of supports* (9th ed.). American Association on Mental Retardation.

Maddux, J. E. (2009). Stopping the "madness": Positive psychology and deconstructing the illness ideology and the DSM. In S. J. Lopez & C. R. Snyder (Eds.), *Oxford handbook of positive psychology* (2nd ed., pp. 61–69). Oxford University Press.

Mazzucchelli, T. G., Kane, R. T., & Rees, C. S. (2010). Behavioral activation interventions for well-being: A meta-analysis. *Journal of Positive Psychology, 5*(2), 105–121.

Meyers, M. C., van Woerkom, M., de Reuver, R., Bakk, Z., & Oberski, D. L. (2015). Enhancing psychological capital and personal growth initiative: Working on strengths or deficiencies? *Journal of Counseling Psychology, 62*(1), 50–62. https://doi.org/10.1037/cou0000050

Niemiec, R. M. (2014). *Mindfulness and character strengths: A practical guide to flourishing.* Hogrefe.

Niemiec, R. M. (2018). *Character strengths interventions: A field-guide for practitioners.* Hogrefe.

Niemiec, R. M. (2023). Mental health and character strengths: the dual role of boosting well-being and reducing suffering. Mental Health and Social Inclusion, Vol. ahead-of-print No. ahead-of-print. https://doi.org/10.1108/MHSI-01-2023-0012

Niemiec, R. M., & Pearce, R. (2021). The practice of character strengths: Unifying definitions, principles, and exploration of what's soaring, emerging, and ripe with potential in science and in practice. *Frontiers in Psychology, 11*, 590220. https://doi.org/10.3389/fpsyg.2020.590220

Niemiec, R. M., Shogren, K. A., & Wehmeyer, M. L. (2017). Character strengths and intellectual and developmental disability: A strengths-based approach from positive psychology. *Education and Training in Autism and Developmental Disabilities, 52*(1), 13–25.

Officer, A., & Shakespeare, T. (2013). The world report on disability and people with intellectual disabilities. *Journal of Policy and Practice in Intellectual Disabilities, 10*(2), 86–88. https://doi.org/10.1111/jppi.12031

Pearce, R. (2018). Be a project motivator: Unlock the secrets of strengths-based project management. Berrett-Koehler Publishers.

Peláez, M. J., Coo, C., & Salanova, M. (2020). Facilitating work engagement and performance through strengths-based micro-coaching: A controlled trial study. *Journal of Happiness Studies: An Interdisciplinary Forum on Subjective Well-Being, 21*(4), 1265–1284. https://doi.org/10.1007/s10902-019-00127-5

Rashid, T., & Ostermann, R. F. (2009). Strength-based assessment in clinical practice. *Journal of Clinical Psychology: In Session, 65*(5), 488–498.

Rashid, T., & Seligman, M. E. P. (2019). *Positive psychotherapy: Clinician manual.* Oxford University Press.

Rogers, C. (1961). *On becoming a person.* Houghton Mifflin.

Rozin, P., & Royzman, E. B. (2001). Negativity bias, negativity dominance, and contagion. *Personality and Social Psychology Review, 5*(4), 296–320.

Saleebey, D. (1992). *The strengths perspective in social work practice.* Longman.

Saleebey, D. (1996). The strengths perspective in social work practice: Extension and cautions. *Social Work, 41*(3), 296–305.

Seligman, M. E. P. (1999). The president's address. *American Psychologist, 54*, 559–562.

Shogren, K. A. (2013). *Self-determination and transition planning.* Paul H. Brookes Publishing.

Smith, E. J. (2006). The strength-based counseling model. *The Counseling Psychologist, 34*(1), 13–79.

Steimer, A., & Mata, A. (2016). Motivated implicit theories of personality: My weaknesses will go away, but my strengths are here to stay. *Personality and Social Psychology Bulletin, 42*(4), 415–429. https://doi.org/10.1177/0146167216629437

Teffert, D. A. (2009). The savant syndrome: An extraordinary condition. A synopsis: Past, present, future. *Philosophical Transactions of the Royal Society of London. Series B, Biological Sciences, 364*(1522), 1351–1357. https://doi.org/10.1098/rstb.2008.0326

van Woerkom, M., Mostert, K., Els, C., Bakker, A. B., de Beer, L., & Rothmann, S. (2016). Strengths use and deficit correction in organizations: Development and validation of a questionnaire. *European Journal of Work and Organizational Psychology.* https://doi.org/10.1080/1359432X.2016.1193010

Vertilo, V., & Gibson, J. M. (2014). Influence of character strengths on mental health stigma. *Journal of Positive Psychology, 9*, 266–275. https://doi.org/10.1111/1467-9450.00242

Wehmeyer, M. L. (2005). Self-determination and individuals with severe disabilities: Reexamining meanings and misinterpretations. *Research and Practice in Severe Disabilities, 30*, 113–120.

Wehmeyer, M. L. (Ed.). (2013). *The Oxford handbook of positive psychology and disability*. Oxford University Press.

Wehmeyer, M. L. (2020). Strengths-based approaches to disability, the supports paradigm, and the importance of the supports intensity scales. *Revista Educação Especial, 33*, 1–14.

Wehmeyer, M. L., & Little, T. D. (2013). Self-determination. In M. L. Wehmeyer (Ed.), The Oxford handbook of positive psychology and disability (pp. 116–136). Oxford University Press.

Welch, D., Grossaint, K., Reid, K., & Walker, C. (2014). Strengths-based leadership development: Insights from expert coaches. *Consulting Psychology Journal: Practice and Research, 66*(1), 20–37. https://doi.org/10.1037/cpb0000002

World Health Organization. (2021). *Disability and health*. https://www.who.int/news-room/fact-sheets/detail/disability-and-health. Accessed on 23 Sept 2022.

Wright, B. A., & Lopez, S. J. (2009). Widening the diagnostic focus: A case for including human strengths and environmental resources. In S. J. Lopez & C. R. Snyder (Eds.), *Oxford handbook of positive psychology* (2nd ed., pp. 71–487). Oxford University Press.

Chapter 2
Character Strengths: Finding Ability, Well-Being, and Cultivating Resilience

The Concepts

In 2004, a landmark achievement occurred in the social sciences: A classification of character strengths, rooted in science, was unleashed to the world (Peterson & Seligman, 2004). This consensual nomenclature (i.e., "common language") of positive qualities was the result of a 3-year collaboration among more than 50 scientists. The starting point was inquiry: What is best about human beings? What are the positive traits that are part of all humans? What brings a human being to experience a full life, a good life, a meaningful life?

The scientists investigated these questions in several ways:

- Examination of texts on virtues, strengths, positive qualities, including the major writings from each of the most popular world religions, ancient philosophers (e.g., Aristotle), and those who wrote virtue catalogues (e.g., Benjamin Franklin) (Dahlsgaard et al., 2005; Peterson & Seligman, 2004).
- Examination of the research literatures on strengths, virtues, and related areas, for example, moral psychology and developmental psychology (Peterson & Seligman, 2004).
- Construction of psychometrically reliable and valid measurement tools (for adults and youth) to assess character strengths, and administer these across the globe to a diverse array of people across the six major continents (Park et al., 2006; Peterson & Seligman, 2004).
- Traveled to remote cultures, including the Maasai tribal people in Kenya and the Inuit people in Northern Greenland, to inquire and discuss the possible presence and expression of the emerging list of universal character strengths in their culture and ways to cultivate, enable, and inhibit their expression (Biswas-Diener, 2006).

R. M. Niemiec, D. Tomasulo, *Character Strengths and Abilities Within Disabilities*, Positive Psychology and Disability Series,
https://doi.org/10.1007/978-3-031-36294-1_2

Table 2.1 Criteria for 24 character strengths (Peterson & Seligman, 2004)

Character strengths criteria	Definition of criteria
Ubiquitous or universal	The trait is present in people across the planet, namely, the six major continents, and is not bound to a particular culture or country
Measurable	The trait can be accurately assessed in people using a straightforward self-report instrument that demonstrates good psychometrics
Fulfilling	The trait contributes to various fulfillments that constitute a good life for oneself and others
Morally valued	The trait is valued in its own right, even in the absence of obvious beneficial outcomes
Does not diminish others	The display of the strength does not diminish others, rather it more likely results in a win-win for those around the person using the strength
Nonfelicitous opposites	A linguistic test to ensure the opposite of the positive trait is also not positive but in most cases, a negative
Trait-like	The strength manifests in a range of actions across situations and time
Distinctiveness	The strength is distinct from other positive traits in the VIA classification and cannot be decomposed into them
Paragons	The strength is embodied in consensual exemplars or culturally observed role models
Prodigies	The existence of some young people who strongly display this strength
Selective absence	There are people who show a complete lack of the strength in some situations
Institutions and rituals	The larger society provides rituals or mechanisms for display or sustaining the strength, this includes institutional rules, roles, and norms

- Establishment of strengths criteria to evaluate and scrutinize each candidate character strength (Peterson & Seligman, 2004). See Table 2.1 for 12 criteria and definitions. For example, it is important that a character strength not diminish others when it is used and that it is fulfilling in and of itself.

Each of the areas of scientific investigation just bulleted—and each of the criteria—have continued to be studied and expanded as the science of character strengths has continued to evolve in the subsequent two decades.

The result of this rigorous approach was the VIA Classification, which contains 24 character strengths nesting under 6 universal virtues, found across religions and ancient philosophies, and standing the test of time as being relevant and important over the centuries and for today's world. For example, curiosity and creativity are wisdom strengths, honesty and perseverance are courage strengths, and kindness and social intelligence are humanity strengths. See Table 2.2 for the full VIA Classification with shortened descriptions.

Since the release of the VIA Classification in 2004, several-hundred studies have been conducted across the globe, amounting to a wide array of knowledge and practices on character strengths. These insights have culminated into a multifaceted *definition* of character strengths as positive personality traits that:

1. Reflect core identity.
2. Produce positive outcomes for oneself and others.
3. Contribute to the collective good (Niemiec, 2018).

Table 2.2 VIA Classification of character strengths and virtues (Peterson & Seligman, 2004)

Virtue	Character strength	Description
Wisdom	Creativity	Being original; seeing/doing things in new ways
	Curiosity	Exploring; seeking novelty; open to experiences
	Judgment	Critical thinking; rational-minded; thinking things through
	Love of learning	Mastering new skills and topics; building knowledge
	Perspective	Providing wise counsel; taking a big picture view
Courage	Bravery	Facing fears, threats, or challenges; speaking up for what's right
	Perseverance	Persisting; finishing what is started; overcoming obstacles
	Honesty	Telling the truth; being authentic; being sincere
	Zest	Being energetic; enthusiastic; doing things wholeheartedly
Humanity	Love	Being genuine; showing warmth; valuing close relationships
	Kindness	Being generous; caring; compassionate; nice and friendly
	Social intelligence	Being aware of feelings and motives of self/others; acting accordingly
Justice	Teamwork	Being loyal; contributing to group efforts
	Fairness	Acting justly; not letting feelings bias decisions
	Leadership	Organizing a group to get things done; positively guiding others
Temperance	Forgiveness	Being merciful; accepting others' shortcomings; letting go of hurts
	Humility	Being modest; placing attention on others; not bragging
	Prudence	Being careful about choices; cautious; not taking undue risks
	Self-regulation	Being self-controlled; disciplined; managing impulses and emotions
Transcendence	Appreciation of beauty/excellence	Experiencing awe, wonder, admiration, elevation
	Gratitude	Being thankful for the good in life; sharing thanks; feeling blessed
	Hope	Being optimistic; positive; future-minded; expecting the best
	Humor	Being playful, seeing the lighter side, bringing smiles to others
	Spirituality	Searching for meaning; feeling purpose in life; connecting with the sacred

This means that character strengths, respectively, help to answer the questions: Who am I? How might I build better relationships, achieve more, get healthier, or tap into more meaning in life? How might I become a better person, support my family or community, or contribute more to the social good?

Building off this definition, we examine five character strengths principles. These central concepts lay a foundation to facilitate an understanding of the depth and nuances of character strengths.

These collective works—the VIA Classification of strengths and virtues, the VIA Survey measurement tool, and the initiation of the classic text *Character Strengths and Virtues* (Peterson & Seligman, 2004)—were put forth by the nonprofit, VIA Institute on Character, founded in 2000. To learn more about the VIA Institute, see Appendix 1.

Character Strengths Are Dimensional

In a world filled with black or white, all or none thinking, and diagnostic systems for categorizing illness, disorders, diseases, and disabilities (*ICD-11* and *DSM-5*), there also exist many phenomena resting on dimensions. Strengths of character are some of these phenomena, as character strengths are expressed in degrees. A person is not a creative person all the time nor does creativity fully capture who they are, rather a person is "more or less" creative based on the situation they are in and the individual and interpersonal variables at play (Miller, 2013; Niemiec, 2018; Peterson & Seligman, 2004).

Character Is Plural

One of the field-changing insights to emerge from the science of character strengths is that character is plural (Peterson, 2006). This means that character is individualized and unique to each person who has their own constellation of character strengths and expresses them in unique ways. Plurality approaches say that people are not simply brave or loving, curious or fair; rather, people show a variation and combination of character strengths that make up a rich and personal tapestry. As situations become increasingly challenging or complex, the constellations of character strengths expressed increases. For example, a person who is sipping coffee while gazing at trees in their backyard may mostly be using their appreciation of beauty and curiosity strengths, while the person who has been fired from their job and wants to handle the situation magnanimously, needs to call upon a range of character strengths. This person may turn to the self-regulation of their emotions, prudence for planning new career possibilities, humility to stay centered amidst the stress, self-forgiveness and self-kindness, social intelligence with colleagues as they make the transition, and bravery, curiosity, and love of learning to face new frontiers, to name a few.

Character Is Expressed in Situations

While character strengths are experienced cognitively, emotionally, and volitionally within, the outward expression and validity of that expression occurs in words and behaviors. These expressions vary by context. An individual may express different degrees of character strengths at work, school, home, and community; in this way the frequency (how often the strength is expressed), the duration (how long the strength is expressed), and the intensity (how strong the strength is expressed) will shift based on the domain. Further, each situation within that domain will elicit subtle or obvious changes. For example, one person may use their character strength of love at work by hugging their work colleague in a situation in which their colleague shares about an upsetting weekend; and 1 h later that same person uses their strength of love with their boss by being warm and friendly as they speak about the day's agenda. That same person then might go home that evening and express their strength of love with their partner by cooking the partner's favorite dinner. Each situation within each domain of life is different due to the setting, context, the different people who are present, the psychological makeup of each person present (their mood, personality, etc.), and the history of the interactions, and thereby the combination of character strengths and the degrees to which they are expressed will vary.

All 24 Character Strengths Matter

Each character strength has been studied over the decades and has been associated with a range of positive variables (Peterson & Seligman, 2004). For example, hope and zest are the character strengths found repeatedly to have the strongest links with happiness (e.g., Park et al., 2004; Proctor et al., 2009), while perseverance is critical for achievement (e.g., Lounsbury et al., 2009) and other variables such as positive emotions, engagement, meaning, and positive relationships each have their highest character strengths correlates (Wagner et al., 2019). These associations for character strengths are not guarantees for certain outcomes and there will be variability within each person and situation, nevertheless, there is an increased chance of the positive benefits. In addition to the connection between character strengths and positive outcomes, the working theory is that all human beings have the capacity to express all 24 of these character strengths to some degree (Biswas-Diener, 2006; Niemiec, 2018; Peterson & Seligman, 2004). In this way, for each individual, each character strength becomes vitally important; the person may need to rely upon their prudence and self-regulation in one situation and upon creativity, curiosity, and perspective in the situation that follows.

Character Strengths Can Be Developed

For many readers, this theoretical concept is "saving the best for last." All character strengths can be mindfully targeted and increased or improved upon (Niemiec, 2018; Pang & Ruch, 2019). Research on personality traits shows that individuals' personality is more malleable than originally thought and personality change does not have to be gradual (Blackie et al., 2014; Hudson & Fraley, 2015; Roberts et al., 2017). There are many factors that can bring forth changes in personality, one of which is referred to as deliberate interventions (e.g., Borghans et al., 2008). Intervention studies are showing that deliberate attempts to bring forth change in personality (of which character strengths are part) can have a positive impact (Yeager et al., 2014; Hudson & Fraley, 2015; Roberts et al., 2017). Individuals may decide to focus on one of their signature strengths and expand upon it (Gander et al., 2013) or they may wish to improve upon one of their lower character strengths in their profile (Proyer et al., 2015). These emerging empirical findings over the last two decades provide encouragement for not only practitioners and consumers aiming to self-develop, but also for practitioners to better help their clients, patients, employees, and students.

The Science

At the time of this writing, there have been more than 900 studies published on character strengths involving the VIA Inventory and/or VIA Classification (VIA Institute, 2023); this number excludes the tens of thousands of studies across the individual character strengths, such as the vast literature on creativity, leadership, spirituality, gratitude, and so on. This catapult of research encompasses a range of studies that examine correlates, causes, populations, contexts, grouping of character strengths, and different assessment measures of character strengths.

The areas most studied are the workplace and education. In the workplace, character strengths are associated with a variety of well-being (Littman-Ovadia & Steger, 2010) and workplace performance benefits (Harzer et al., 2021), as well as more prosocial behavior (Freidlin & Littman-Ovadia, 2020) and better workplace climate (van Woerkom & Meyers, 2014). In the education context, character strengths interventions are consistently associated with well-being benefits across studies (e.g., Oppenheimer et al., 2014; Proctor et al., 2011; Quinlan et al., 2014), and discussion of implementation across schools and deeply within the fabrics of schools has been successfully applied (Coppley & Niemiec, 2021; White & Waters, 2014). There are a number of other domains of living that have examined character strengths. Table 2.3 offers a sampling of domains in which character strengths have been applied and denotes one example of a study in each domain and its findings.

Another lens by which to parse the hundreds of studies is to consider two large buckets—a bucket of studies relating to building the many kinds of well-being and

Table 2.3 A sampling of character strengths studies across domains of life functioning

Domain of Life	Reference (limiting to one)	Key finding
Work	Bakker and van Wingerden (2020)	Randomized study showing strengths training increases work engagement, personal resources, and strengths use
School	Haslip et al. (2019)	Examined strengths-spotting in examples of teachers and children and finding connections with empathy, affection, friendship, helping behavior, and speaking positively
Positive relationships	Kashdan et al. (2017)	Recognition and appreciation of character strengths in one's relationship partner predicted greater relationship commitment, satisfaction, intimacy, and needs met
Relationships—friendships	Wagner (2018)	This study found that certain character strengths (honesty, humor, kindness, fairness) were most desirable and important for peers to have in a friend, while other character strengths were more connected with higher peer acceptance
Leisure	Wagner et al. (2021)	Character strengths profiles were significantly associated with the leisure domain and this was connected with flourishing
Parenting	Allen et al. (2022)	Strengths-based parenting was connected to growth, positive reappraisal, and emotional processing
Health	Proyer et al. (2013)	Character strengths show strong connections across numerous health behaviors, especially self-regulation, curiosity, appreciation of beauty, gratitude, hope, and humor
Spirituality	Niemiec et al. (2020)	Explores the evidence for integrating spirituality and character strengths and proposes a theoretical model and practices for the mutual synergy of character strengths and secular spirituality
Earth/ environment	Merino et al. (2020)	Character strengths were strongly connected with nature connection, especially appreciation of beauty, followed by love of learning and curiosity

a bucket of studies relating to understanding, managing, and/or overcoming adversity. For the former, character strengths are causal factors for happiness and are connected with physical health, positive relationships, achievement, and meaning in life. For the latter, character strengths are important for handling stress and conflict, from everyday tensions to major life events. Theorizing has proposed that optimal thriving in life requires both the well-being/opportunity functions of character strengths and adversity functions (Niemiec, 2020). Table 2.4 offers a small sampling of character strengths studies across these two buckets.

The science of character strengths extends well beyond the outcome-focused tables in this chapter, such as measurement of character strengths, further theoretical articles (e.g., overuse and underuse of strengths), factor analysis studies, qualitative studies, interview studies, case examples, studies of strengths dynamics, and research in specific populations. Some of these are covered in other chapters, for

Table 2.4 A sampling of character strengths studies across well-being and adversity areas

	References (limiting to one)	Key finding
Well-being area		
Inner peace	Cherif et al. (2022)	The character strengths most connected to two different types of inner peace were hope, followed by zest and gratitude (primary), while secondary character strengths connected with inner peace were forgiveness and spirituality
Happiness	Proyer et al. (2013)	Across multiple studies, the character strengths most connected with happiness—and causal for happiness in the study here—are zest, hope, love, curiosity, and gratitude (although this particular study replaced love with humor)
Positive emotions	Wagner et al. (2019)	The character strengths most connected to positive emotions (per self-report and informant report) were zest, hope, and humor
Autonomy	Harzer (2016)	A comprehensive review found the character strengths most connected with autonomy were honesty, bravery, and perspective
Mindfulness	Pang and Ruch (2019)	The character strengths most connected with total mindfulness and most mindfulness skills were hope, bravery, curiosity, zest, and social intelligence
Meaning	Peterson et al. (2007)	The character strengths most associated with meaning were spirituality, gratitude, hope, zest, and curiosity
Achievement	Villacís et al. (2021)	Character strengths showed positive associations with academic performance among undergraduate students
Healthy self-care	Weziak-Bialowolska et al. (2023)	The character strengths most connected with healthy self-care activities and routines were zest, hope, self-regulation, curiosity, and gratitude
Adversity area		
Grief	Blanchard et al. (2021)	Character strengths showed stability across three time points among adults experiencing a loss; some strengths were associated with less impairment and depression
Anxiety	Freidlin et al. (2017)	Individuals with (and without) social anxiety disorder were able to be correctly sorted (with nearly 90% accuracy) based on their patterns of character strengths overuse and underuse
Depression	Schutte and Malouff (2019)	Meta-analysis revealing that randomized-controlled trials using the intervention "use a signature strength in a new way" leads to greater well-being, flourishing, strengths levels, and less depression
Coping in youth	Toback et al. (2016)	Randomized study creating interventions linking the top character strengths with coping strategies among psychiatrically hospitalized youth and finding sustained benefits to self-efficacy and self-esteem
Chronic pain	Graziosi et al. (2020)	Of the 24 character strengths, zest was the highest associated with pain self-efficacy and a zest intervention boosted this variable and the capacity to function despite pain
Trauma	Peterson et al. (2008)	The more traumatic events reported by an individual, the higher the character strengths scores (with a few exceptions)

(continued)

Table 2.4 (continued)

	References (limiting to one)	Key finding
Natural disasters	Duan et al. (2015)	Among people in China who experienced a natural disaster, there was a strong relationship between character strengths/virtues and resilience and the former contributed strongly to post-traumatic growth
War and terrorism	Shoshani and Slone (2016)	Among more than 1000 adolescents exposed to long periods of war, terrorism, and political conflict, numerous character strengths were found to negatively relate to psychiatric symptoms

example, measurement in Chap. 3, overuse/underuse in Chap. 6, and studies of particular populations in Chaps. 4, 5, 6, 7, and 8.

The Practice

How is a practitioner—whoever the individual is that they are supporting—to use a strengths-based approach? There are seemingly infinite ways a person could generically or deeply deploy any kind of strength to help others. In addition, there is a wide range of intensity in that application, ranging from very light intensity (e.g., "Can I get you a cup of coffee?" or at the end of a meeting, "Tell me about one of your strengths?") to high intensity (e.g., systematic integration of strengths into all actions in a meeting). To propose an operational approach for practitioners based in the emerging science and best practices, Niemiec and Pearce (2021) zeroed in on the character strengths practitioners' optimal approach. They proposed the following seven core elements to serve as the definition of a *character strengths-based approach*:

1. *Educates*: The practitioner teaches about character strengths, explains their rationale and importance, corrects misconceptions (e.g., strengths are happiology; or strengths involve ignoring weaknesses), and offers questions and interventions for character strengths use.
2. *Embodies*: The practitioner embodies character strengths in their approach, serving as a role model for character strengths use, thus displaying character strengths awareness, exploration, and application use as they interact with the client.
3. *Energizes*: The practitioner uplifts and fuels the person out of autopilot tendencies, entrapped mental and behavioral routines, and strengths blindness (Biswas-Diener et al., 2011) patterns.
4. *Empowers*: The practitioner focuses on character strengths to help people move from what's wrong to what's strong *and/or* helps them use what's strong to overcome what's wrong (Niemiec, 2023).
5. *Manages adversity*: The practitioner squarely acknowledges problems and struggles—and when appropriate for the context/relationship, explores this suffering

using strengths, offers strategies as to how character strengths can confront, manage, or overcome adversity; and strikes a balance of not getting lost in problems nor allows the positive to be squashed out (Niemiec, 2020).

6. *Connects*: The practitioner knows that positive core qualities are likened to connective tissue helping people to relate and connect with one another. Thus, the practitioner uses character strengths to connect with the client and empower the client to further connect with others, with the world, and with themselves.
7. *Cultivates seeds*: The practitioner realizes the benefits of an orientation involving cultivating seeds, not just plucking weeds (the negative). Rather than engaging only in a prescriptive approach, the descriptive language around character strengths is prioritized to build awareness, to explore, and to help the client grow toward positive action (Linkins et al., 2015; Niemiec, 2014).

These are core descriptors of a character strengths-based approach, and they are also a framing of many of the core actions of a character strengths-based practitioner. Establishing a character strengths approach and deploying it with clients is a way to infuse energy into oneself as the helper but also into the client. The practitioner is energizing oneself with one's best naturally occurring qualities and is bringing that energy to the client or student with discussions, education, and empowerment and thereby encouraging them to tap into their energizing qualities. This is viewed as the **E = mc2 Model** because with this focus on "energy," one can consider how the first letters of the first words of the seven elements map into Einstein's famous equation on energy, $E = mc^2$, as a way to recollect these seven elements (starting with 4 E's, the m, and the squared c's).

While this is not meant to be an exhaustive list, it offers a useful framework for practitioners to move forward as they work with any client using character strengths.

Interventions

The number of character strengths interventions are vast, however, the number of character strengths interventions studied in gold standard studies (i.e., randomized, double-blind, placebo-controlled trials) is far less. That said, meta-analyses of strengths interventions have been positive (e.g., Bates-Krakoff et al., 2022; Ghielen et al., 2017; Schutte & Malouff, 2019). These studies show that strengths can lead to a positive behavior change (Bates-Krakoff et al., 2022), an increase in well-being and decrease in depression (Schutte & Malouff, 2019), and higher work engagement, personal growth, and group/team benefits (Ghielen et al., 2017). Despite these being positive comprehensive reviews, more studies are needed particularly those that focus on behavioral change. Niemiec (2018) offers guidelines for practitioners on categorizing character strengths interventions encouraging practitioners to look to gold-standard studies and also to cautiously look beyond these to studies that have a scientific or theoretical base for the construction of the intervention; this may include interventions adapted from quality studies and interventions that are one component of a larger intervention program that has been shown to be effective.

Along these lines, we share five interventions that have an evidence-base *and* that practitioners report are highly beneficial for clients. With each intervention, a real-world example of a client or student of ours is offered.

Take the VIA *Inventory of Strengths (*VIA *Survey)*: This assessment is also a positive intervention. Taking the test and reviewing the results can lead the person to a deeper self-understanding, can break through negativity mindsets, and can help pave a path toward healthy future action.

When Isaiah was asked about his reactions to his results, he explained that curiosity was his highest strength and that at first he was surprised by this as he had never viewed his curiosity as a strength of his character. Upon reflecting, he observed that curiosity is part of nearly everything in his life. It is in his asking his supervisor questions each day so he can do his job well. It is in his exploring of solutions with his relationship partner when they have a conflict. It is in his interest in curiously wandering about social media posts and Internet sites. It is also in his quest for knowledge as he looks up DIY videos when something breaks down in his home.

Affirm and value character strengths: It is one thing to take a measure of well-being or character strengths, but it is quite another thing to truly acknowledge and appreciate one's best qualities. This involves linking character strengths to actions taken at home and work/school. It also involves considering why character strengths are of value and of meaning for oneself.

Micah had a personality style that was quite negative and pessimistic. She was encouraged by her employer to take the VIA Survey. After reviewing her highest five character strengths, she journaled about two questions for each strength: How do I see this strength in myself? Why do I value this strength in myself? She approached the activity very thoughtfully and strategically. As a result, she could not believe what happened next: She wrote 20 pages of examples of her top 5 strengths! She wrote about how she uses each one, in small ways, with her family, her friends, and co-workers. She explored how her highest strengths were of great value to her in persevering to get promotions at work so that she could provide financially for her family and she wrote about how her creativity and spirituality strengths fuel herself with energy, ideas, and connections and thus helping her feel happier.

Expand and use signature strengths: This intervention advances the previous two. Using signature strengths in new ways has been examined in multiple studies which collectively led to a meta-analysis of those intervention studies, finding signature strengths use led to greater flourishing, life satisfaction, and use of strengths, and less depression (Schutte & Malouff, 2019).

Jennifer was someone who struggled with depression her whole life. While she had tried many avenues, she was perseverant and would not give up. She came upon character strengths and set forth a plan to use her highest strengths each day. Each morning she mapped out at least one new way she would use one strength that day—while at the grocery store, when with her daughter, or when looking for a new job. After a couple weeks, she observed that she felt as if the roof above her had opened up and she was no longer boxed in. She could now see the light shining above and the vibrant blue sky. She felt more free to be herself.

Practice strengths-spotting: The practice of seeing strengths in people can be applied to oneself and any person, known and unknown, in one's life. The 3-step SEA model—spot/label the strength, explain/give rationale for the strength noticed, appreciate/share the importance of what is observed—can be a useful framework for strengths-spotting. Strengths-spotting is a skill that improves as we practice. Noah had this to say about his strengths-spotting practice:

> Once I put on my "strengths goggles," there is no stopping me. I can see these character strengths in each person I come in contact with. This applies to the bagger at the grocery store, the support person at the shoe store, my child who has just come home from school, my grandmother when she calls me, my neighbor I see when I am out for a walk, and even the various characters in the TV series I am watching. The hardest part is seeing the strengths in myself when I am using them, but I am improving on this.

Strengths alignment: An important finding in strengths work is that your top strengths can be consciously and successfully aligned with tasks and activities in daily life. Research in a controlled trial found that workers who deliberately connected their signature strengths with their work tasks experienced higher life satisfaction and work that was a calling in life (Harzer & Ruch, 2016).

Amir, a high level marketing executive, was feeling burned out in his work. He engaged in the activity of listing his top five character strengths, listing five of the main tasks he did most days at work, and then looked for ways to align these two lists; in other words to bring at least one strength into each of his main work tasks. For the work activity of leading a daily morning team meeting, Amir decided he would bring gratitude into the meeting by making a point to express appreciation (and rationale for the appreciation) to one teammate, to his organization, or to his field each day. For his work activity of making a check-in client phone call, he decided he would use his strength of curiosity to spend more time exploring and asking his client questions as opposed to only spouting out advice. For his activity of creating marketing presentations, he would turn to his strength of judgment/critical thinking to ensure his slides had a strong research backing and rationale for use, as he knew the management team valued that. After infusing these and other character strengths into his work, Amir felt more energized and fulfilled.

For a more exhaustive discussion of research-based interventions, see *Character Strengths Interventions* (Niemiec, 2018).

Self-Practice

Practitioners, educators, managers, parents, and other professionals who want to apply or are applying character strengths with others are strongly encouraged to practice using character strengths with themselves. This will help the practitioner come from a foundation of strength and understanding to support others. We offer four adages that support this tenet.

Know thyself: Self-awareness is the essential starting point. We all have extensive degrees of internal strengths blindness, therefore, cultivating an awareness and understanding of all of our 24 character strengths, and how they have, do, or could manifest, is the initial personal work.

Walk the talk or practice what you preach: Few things are more inauthentic than the person who talks and advises others but does not go to any effort to apply practices to themselves. The personal work one does with character strengths can directly lead to greater ease and savvy in applying the character strengths to help others. Not only does the helper better understand how to navigate strengths (as they already did it for themselves), but the helper is coming from a stronger position—a foundation laid of strengths wisdom and growth.

Who we are is what we repeatedly do: This variation of an Aristotle saying points to a reality that what we fasten as a routine in our life is a reflection of our identity. If we practice (even mindlessly) being angry or aggressive then that becomes a significant part of who we are. If we practice courage and kindness then that becomes who we are.

The only practice that matters is the one you do: This variation of a Gottlieb (2012) expression points to the importance of action. We can study and discuss many ideas, we can wait for new research studies to arise, and we can reflect on a myriad of practices, but in the end, there is only one practice that is relevant—it is the one that you actually put into action.

Types of Practice

A natural next question then emerges—how shall I practice? We offer four general ways a practice can be initiated, advanced, and maintained for oneself or one's clients/students:

Formal practice: having a regular routine—same time each day. A person might journal about their character strengths use at the end of each day, use their curiosity each morning while having breakfast with a family member, or pause at lunch each day to reflect on one's signature strengths and how they might be used at work the remainder of the day.

Practice in routines: considering one's daily routines and habits (e.g., taking a shower, brewing coffee, making one's bed) and posing two questions: Which character strength(s) am I naturally using—no matter how small the amount of strength—in this routine? Which character strength would I like to use to bring more energy into this routine? A person might realize they are using self-regulation because they never forget to brush their teeth every morning, thus reflecting some degree of discipline and self-management. They might then plan to bring in more kindness and prudence to their habit as they brush their teeth more slowly, carefully, and gently. This approach supports the person in making character strengths a deliberate part of life.

External cues practice: setting up external reminders to use strengths. With this practice, one uses the environment as a prompt to turn to one's internal qualities. This is important because it is easy to slip into mindless routines and to forget about one's strengths. Therefore, with a cue that is personally set up, one can then turn to a signature strength in that moment. For example, one might say that whenever a "bell sound" naturally occurs or whenever one notices another person smile, then that is the cue to remember to turn to one signature strength. Likewise, a person might place sticky notes, pictures, or other stickers in different places of one's work and home environment to cue oneself to return to one's strengths in that situation.

Informal practice: using character strengths when one needs them. Conflicts, unexpected stressors, and internal problems arise in small and large doses throughout the weeks. The more one has tapped into the preceding types of practice, the more equipped and empowered one is to use character strengths in those difficult moments. This is when the practice of character strengths "pays off" and benefits the person offering them a perspective of greater resilience.

Future Directions

From a basic research perspective, studies in character strengths have risen substantially since the advent of the VIA Inventory/VIA Survey and VIA Classification, far beyond expectations in a way that is rarely seen in the field of psychology. Similarly, the response from practitioners in different fields—especially the organizational, educational, and coaching contexts—has been filled with enthusiasm, creativity, and an eagerness to develop applications. However, one of the bridges between these two groups—the bridge of randomized-controlled trials of character strengths interventions—has been less prolific.

Therefore, our strongest suggestion for future directions is the examination of the efficacy and effectiveness of character strengths interventions in laboratories and real-life settings. This includes single-session, multi-session, and programmatic studies of character strengths, within multiple settings and for various populations. Further study of how and why character strengths interventions are effective, as well as adaptations that tailor interventions to the unique individual, to relationships between individuals, and to larger social systems to help individuals and groups thrive, would be further advancements.

Key Takeaways

- Character strengths are positive personality traits that reflect core identity, produce positive outcomes for oneself and others, and contribute to the collective good (Niemiec, 2018).
- The VIA Classification of character strengths was a comprehensive landmark achievement in the social sciences and provides a "common language" framework of what is best in human beings.

- The 24 character strengths are trait-like, do not diminish others, are distinct from one another, are fulfilling in and of themselves, are measurable and universal, and have institutions that foster them.
- Character strengths are dimensional, plural, expressed in contexts, and can be developed. All 24 strengths matter. This means there are different outcomes and benefits that emerge from each.
- The scientific studies in character strengths span across contexts and point to two large buckets—benefits for many areas of individual well-being and benefits for many kinds of adversity.
- A character strengths-based approach or character strengths-based practitioner is one who educates on strengths, embodies, energizes, and empowers with strengths, manages adversity, connects, and cultivates seeds of strengths (captured with the $E = mc^2$ acronym).
- There are an extensive array of character strengths interventions that have science-backing and practitioner-enthusiasm, including strengths alignment, spotting, valuing, and use.
- The best character strength practice to use with others is often the one that has been first tested on oneself. Working on one's own character strengths—establishing a formal/informal/routines/cued practice—is foundational and pivotal in order to optimally help others with their strengths.

References

Allen, K. A., Waters, L., Arslan, G., & Prentice, M. (2022). Strength-based parenting and stress-related growth in adolescents: Exploring the role of positive reappraisal, school belonging, and emotional processing during the pandemic. *Journal of Adolescence*. https://doi.org/10.1002/jad.12016

Bakker, A. B., & van Wingerden, J. (2020). Do personal resources and strengths use increase work engagement? The effects of a training intervention. *Journal of Occupational Health Psychology*. https://doi.org/10.1037/ocp0000266

Bates-Krakoff, J., Parente, A., McGrath, R. E., Rashid, T., & Niemiec, R. M. (2022). Are character strength-based positive interventions effective for eliciting positive behavioral outcomes? A meta-analytic review. *International Journal of Wellbeing, 12*(3), 56–80. https://doi.org/10.5502/ijw.v12i3.2111

Biswas-Diener, R. (2006). From the equator to the north pole: A study of character strengths. *Journal of Happiness Studies, 7*, 293–310. https://doi.org/10.1007/s10902-005-3646-8

Biswas-Diener, R., Kashdan, T. B., & Minhas, G. (2011). A dynamic approach to psychological strength development and intervention. *Journal of Positive Psychology, 6*(2), 106–118. https://doi.org/10.1080/17439760.2010.545429

Blackie, L. E. R., Roepke, A. M., Forgeard, M. J. C., Jayawickreme, E., & Fleeson, W. (2014). Act well to be well: The promise of changing personality states to promote well-being. In A. C. Parks & S. Schueller (Eds.), *The Wiley-Blackwell handbook of positive psychological interventions* (pp. 462–474). Wiley-Blackwell.

Blanchard, T., McGrath, R. E., & Jayawickreme. (2021). Resilience in the face of interpersonal loss: The role of character strengths. *Applied Psychology: Health and Well-Being*. https://doi.org/10.1111/aphw.12273

Borghans, L., Duckworth, A. L., Heckman, J. J., & ter Weel, B. (2008). The economics and psychology of personality traits. *Journal of Human Resources, 43*(4), 972–1059. https://doi.org/10.1353/jhr.2008.0017

Cherif, L., Niemiec, R. M., & Wood, V. (2022). Character strengths and inner peace. *International Journal of Wellbeing, 12*(3), 16–34. https://doi.org/10.5502/ijw.v12i3.2195

Coppley, J., & Niemiec, R. M. (2021). Character strengths interventions in education systems. In M. L. Kern & M. L. Wehmeyer (Eds.), *The Palgrave handbook of positive education* (pp. 395–420). Palgrave Macmillan. https://doi.org/10.1007/978-3-030-64537-3_16

Dahlsgaard, K., Peterson, C., & Seligman, M. E. P. (2005). Shared virtue: The convergence of valued human strengths across culture and history. *Review of General Psychology, 9*, 203–213. https://doi.org/10.1037/1089-2680.9.3.203

Duan, W., Guo, P., & Gan, P. (2015). Relationships among trait resilience, virtues, post-traumatic stress disorder, and post-traumatic growth. *PLoS One*. https://doi.org/10.1371/journal.pone.0125707

Freidlin, P., & Littman-Ovadia, H. (2020). Prosocial behavior at work through the lens of character strengths. *Frontiers in Psychology, 10*, Article 3046. https://doi.org/10.3389/fpsyg.2019.03046

Freidlin, P., Littman-Ovadia, H., & Niemiec, R. M. (2017). Positive psychopathology: Social anxiety via character strengths underuse and overuse. *Personality and Individual Differences, 108*, 50–54. https://doi.org/10.1016/j.paid.2016.12.003

Gander, F., Proyer, R. T., Ruch, W., & Wyss, T. (2013). Strength-based positive interventions: Further evidence for their potential in enhancing well-being and alleviating depression. *Journal of Happiness Studies, 14*, 1241–1259. https://doi.org/10.1007/s10902-012-9380-0

Ghielen, S. T. S., van Woerkom, M., & Christina Meyers, M. (2017). Promoting positive outcomes through strengths interventions: A literature review. Journal of Positive Psychology. https://doi.org/10.1080/17439760.2017.1365164

Gottlieb, R. S. (2012). *Spirituality: What it is and why it matters*. Oxford University Press.

Graziosi, M., Yaden, D., Clifton, J., Mikanik, N., & Niemiec, R. M. (2020). A strengths-based approach to chronic pain. *Journal of Positive Psychology*. https://doi.org/10.1080/17439760.2020.1858337

Harzer, C. (2016). The eudaimonics of human strengths: The relations between character strengths and well-being. In J. Vitterso (Ed.), *Handbook of eudaimonic well-being* (pp. 307–322). Springer. https://doi.org/10.1007/978-3-319-42445-3_20

Harzer, C., & Ruch, W. (2016). Your strengths are calling: Preliminary results of a web-based strengths intervention to increase calling. *Journal of Happiness Studies, 17*(6), 2237–2256. https://doi.org/10.1007/s10902-015-9692-y

Harzer, C., Bezuglova, N., & Weber, M. (2021). Incremental validity of character strengths as predictors of job performance beyond general mental ability and the big five. *Frontiers in Psychology, 12*. https://doi.org/10.3389/fpsyg.2021.518369

Haslip, M. J., Allen-Handy, A., & Donaldson, L. (2019). How do children and teachers demonstrate love, kindness and forgiveness? Findings from an early childhood strength-spotting intervention. Early Childhood Education Journal. Advance online publication. https://doi.org/10.1007/s10643-019-00951-7

Hudson, N. W., & Fraley, R. C. (2015). Volitional personality trait change: Can people choose to change their personality traits? *Journal of Personality and Social Psychology, 109*(3), 490–507. https://doi.org/10.1037/pspp0000021

Kashdan, T. B., Blalock, D. V., Young, K. C., Machell, K. A., Monfort, S. S., McKnight, P. E., & Ferssizidis, P. (2017). Personality strengths in romantic relationships: Measuring perceptions of benefits and costs and their impact on personal and relational well-being. *Psychological Assessment*. https://doi.org/10.1037/pas0000464

Linkins, M., Niemiec, R. M., Gillham, J., & Mayerson, D. (2015). Through the strengths lens: A framework for educating the heart. *Journal of Positive Psychology, 10*(1), 64–68

Littman-Ovadia, H., & Steger, M. (2010). Character strengths and well-being among volunteers and employees: Toward an integrative model. *Journal of Positive Psychology, 5*(6), 419–430.

Lounsbury, J. W., Fisher, L. A., Levy, J. J., & Welsh, D. P. (2009). An investigation of character strengths in relation to the academic success of college students. *Individual Differences Research, 7*(1), 52–69.

Merino, A., Valor, C., & Redondo, C. (2020). Connectedness is in my character: The relationship between nature relatedness and character strengths. *Environmental Education Research.* https://doi.org/10.1080/13504622.2020.1825630

Miller, C. B. (2013). *Moral character: An empirical theory.* Oxford University Press.

Niemiec, R. M. (2014). *Mindfulness and character strengths: A practical guide to flourishing.* Hogrefe.

Niemiec, R. M. (2018). *Character strengths interventions: A field-guide for practitioners.* Hogrefe.

Niemiec, R. M. (2020). Six functions of character strengths for thriving at times of adversity and opportunity: A theoretical perspective. *Applied Research in Quality of Life.* https://doi.org/10.1007/s11482-018-9692-2

Niemiec, R. M. (2023). Mental health and character strengths: the dual role of boosting well-being and reducing suffering. Mental Health and Social Inclusion, Vol. ahead-of-print No. ahead-of-print. https://doi.org/10.1108/MHSI-01-2023-0012

Niemiec, R. M., & Pearce, R. (2021). The practice of character strengths: Unifying definitions, principles, and exploration of what's soaring, emerging, and ripe with potential in science and in practice. *Frontiers in Psychology, 11*, 590220. https://doi.org/10.3389/fpsyg.2020.590220

Niemiec, R. M., Russo-Netzer, P., & Pargament, K. I. (2020). The decoding of the human spirit: A synergy of spirituality and character strengths toward wholeness. *Frontiers in Psychology.* https://doi.org/10.3389/fpsyg.2020.02040

Oppenheimer, M. F., Fialkov, C., Ecker, B., & Portnoy, S. (2014). Teaching to strengths: Character education for urban middle school students. *Journal of Character Education, 10*(2), 91–105.

Pang, D., & Ruch, W. (2019). The mutual support model of mindfulness and character strengths. *Mindfulness.* https://doi.org/10.1007/s12671-019-01103-z

Park, N., Peterson, C., & Seligman, M. E. P. (2004). Strengths of character and well-being. *Journal of Social & Clinical Psychology, 23*, 603–619. https://doi.org/10.1521/jscp.23.5.628.50749

Park, N., Peterson, C., & Seligman, M. E. P. (2006). Character strengths in fifty-four nations and the fifty US states. *Journal of Positive Psychology, 1*, 118–129. https://doi.org/10.1080/17439760600619567

Peterson, C. (2006). *A primer in positive psychology.* Oxford University Press.

Peterson, C., & Seligman, M. E. P. (2004). *Character strengths and virtues: A handbook and classification.* Oxford University Press and American Psychological Association.

Peterson, C., Ruch, W., Beerman, U., Park, N., & Seligman, M. E. P. (2007). Strengths of character, orientations to happiness, and life satisfaction. *Journal of Positive Psychology, 2*, 149–156.

Peterson, C., Park, N., Pole, N., D'Andrea, W., & Seligman, M. E. P. (2008). Strengths of character and posttraumatic growth. *Journal of Traumatic Stress, 21*, 214–217.

Proctor, C., Maltby, J., & Linley, P. A. (2009) Strengths use as a predictor of well-being and health-related quality of life. *Journal of Happiness Studies, 10*, 583–630.

Proctor, C., Tsukayama, E., Wood, A. M., Maltby, J., Fox Eades, J., & Linley, P. A. (2011). Strengths gym: The impact of a character strengths-based intervention on the life satisfaction and well-being of adolescents. *Journal of Positive Psychology, 6*(5), 377–388.

Proyer, R. T., Ruch, W., & Buschor, C. (2013). Testing strengths-based interventions: A preliminary study on the effectiveness of a program targeting curiosity, gratitude, hope, humor, and zest for enhancing life satisfaction. *Journal of Happiness Studies, 14*(1), 275–292. https://doi.org/10.1007/s10902-012-9331-9

Proyer, R. T., Gander, F., Wellenzohn, S., & Ruch, W. (2015). Strengths-based positive psychology interventions: A randomized placebo-controlled online trial on long-term effects for a signature strengths vs. a lesser strengths-intervention. *Frontiers in Psychology, 6.* https://doi.org/10.3389/fpsyg.2015.00456

Quinlan, D. M., Swain, N., Cameron, C., & Vella-Brodrick, D. A. (2014). How 'other people matter' in a classroom-based strengths intervention: Exploring interpersonal strategies and classroom outcomes. *Journal of Positive Psychology*. https://doi.org/10.1080/17439760.2014.920407

Roberts, B. W., Luo, J., Briley, D. A., Chow, P. I., Su, R., & Hill, P. L. (2017). A systematic review of personality trait change through intervention. *Psychological Bulletin, 143*(2), 117–141.

Schutte, N. S., & Malouff, J. M. (2019). The impact of signature character strengths interventions: A meta-analysis. *Journal of Happiness Studies, 20*, 1179–1196. https://doi.org/10.1007/s10902-018-9990-2

Shoshani, A., & Slone, M. (2016). The resilience function of character strengths in the face of war and protracted conflict. *Frontiers in Psychology, 6*. https://doi.org/10.3389/fpsyg.2015.02006

Toback, R. L., Graham-Bermann, S., & Patel, P. D. (2016). Outcomes of a character strengths-based intervention on self-esteem and self-efficacy of psychiatrically hospitalized youths. *Psychiatric Services, 67*(5), 574–577. https://doi.org/10.1176/appi.ps.201500021

van Woerkom, M., & Meyers, M. C. (2014). My strengths count! Effects of a strengths-based psychological climate on positive affect and job performance. *Human Resource Management, 54*(1), 81–103.

VIA Institute. (2023). *What the research says about character strengths*. Available at: https://www.viacharacter.org/research/findings. Accessed 2 Jan 2023.

Villacís, J. L., de la Fuente, J., & Naval, C. (2021). Good character at college: The combined role of second-order character strength factors and phronesis motivation in undergraduate academic outcomes. *International Journal of Environmental Research and Public Health, 18*. https://doi.org/10.3390/ijerph18168263

Wagner, L. (2018). Good character is what we look for in a friend: Character strengths are positively related to peer acceptance and friendship quality in early adolescents. *Journal of Early Adolescence*. https://doi.org/10.1177/0272431618791286

Wagner, L., Gander, F., Proyer, R. T., & Ruch, W. (2019). Character strengths and PERMA: Investigating the relationships of character strengths with a multidimensional framework of well-being. *Applied Research in Quality of Life*. https://doi.org/10.1007/s11482-018-9695-z

Wagner, L., Pindeus, L., & Ruch, W. (2021). Character strengths in the life domains of work, education, leisure, and relationships, and their associations with flourishing. *Frontiers in Psychology*. https://doi.org/10.3389/fpsyg.2021.597534

Weziak-Bialowolska, D., Bialowolski, P., & Niemiec, R. M. (2023). Character strengths and health-related quality of life in a large international sample: A cross-sectional analysis. *Journal of Research in Personality, 103*. https://doi.org/10.1016/j.jrp.2022.104338

White, M. A., & Waters, L. E. (2014). A case study of 'The Good School:' Examples of use of Peterson's strengths-based approach with students. *Journal of Positive Psychology*. https://doi.org/10.1080/17439760.2014.920408

Yeager, D. S., Johnson, R., Spitzer, B. J., Trzesniewski, K. H., Powers, J., & Dweck, C. S. (2014). The far-reaching effects of believing people can change: Implicit theories of personality shape stress, health, and achievement during adolescence. *Journal of Personality and Social Psychology, 106*(6), 867–884. https://doi.org/10.1037/a0036335

Part II
Character Strengths for Specific Disabilities

The chapters in Part II focus on a wide range of disabilities, each with their dedicated analysis, research, and practical considerations and each using the lens of character strengths throughout.

We turn our attention first (Chap. 3) to intellectual/developmental disabilities (IDD) and autism spectrum disorders and explore seven principles important for considering character strengths with these populations. Research on character strengths has focused on the assessment of people with IDD, the character strengths of staff who support them, and the character strengths of sub-populations—who may or may not always fit in this category—such as people with autism. Emerging research is focusing on programmatic outcomes of applying character strengths to people with IDD. The many levels of assessment and intervention are reviewed, with an emphasis on strategies and examples with strengths-spotting. Creating adaptations of existing evidenced-based programs and individualized education plans (IEPs) (and individualized strengths plans; ISPs) are discussed and exemplified.

Chapter 4 highlights the infusion of character strengths into attention-deficit/hyperactivity disorder (ADHD). While a household term and discussed in volumes of scientific studies across the globe, the integration of character strengths has been comparatively nonexistent. We review the scholarly work that has been initiated and offer theoretical extension from character science to ADHD and offer a range of compelling interventions to integrate into existing treatment for ADHD and to serve as potential standalone areas of focus.

Chapter 5 explores trauma, posttraumatic growth, and resilience. Several concepts such as the disability paradox and the resilience paradox are discussed. A handful of studies looking at character strengths and trauma are reviewed. The transformative potential of character strengths, particularly the character strength of hope, is reviewed and exemplified with case examples.

In Chap. 6, we explore the category of psychiatric disability starting with a wide lens in terms of the general patterns in which psychological frameworks have been limited in view and the lack of salutogenic frameworks. We examine research studies that have shown character strengths to have a buffering effect for mental problems and the dual role of character strengths to both enhance well-being and reduce suffering. The overuse, underuse, and optimal-use of character strengths is explored from a conceptual and scientific perspective. A range of practices are explored from general approaches (e.g., intake and treatment planning procedures) to specific character strengths that might be targeted to specific interventions such as the tempering effect and the towing effect.

We then turn to physical and medical disorders in Chap. 7. As the range of conditions here could fill multiple series of textbooks, we give most attention to conditions in which character strengths have received scientific attention. For example, chronic pain, heart disease, and COVID-19 have received several studies. In the practice section, we prioritize the increasing of physical health and the five pillars of health through character strengths practices. We also discuss managing disease and supporting healthcare/medical professions by reducing burnout through strength interventions.

Chapter 3
Intellectual/Developmental Disabilities, Autism Spectrum Disorder, and Character Strengths

The Concepts

> Moving forward, we recommend the [intellectual/developmental disability] field expand its focus beyond the assessment and remediation of deficits to approaches that give priority to the study and practice of character strengths in assessment and intervention (p. 22). Niemiec et al. (2017) Education and Training in Autism and Developmental Disabilities

Positive change toward strengths has been evolving in the intellectual/developmental disability (herein IDD) field over the last few decades. Greater emphasis is being placed on the individual and their needs, desires, and strengths; systems are slowly improving in looking at the positive in each person; professionals are implementing alternative questions and activities that go beyond a deficit-correction approach. Yet the emphasis on character strengths—in comparison with strengths of skill, of interest, and of resources—is not yet widely implemented.

Turning briefly to the science, a systematic review of the positive psychology and intellectual disability literature was conducted and 13 positive psychology constructs (and 22 measures) were identified. The most common constructs were

Clarification: In this chapter, the term intellectual/developmental disability (IDD) is frequently used. IDD is not a one-size-fits-all, discrete condition, for example, while Down syndrome is a common cause of intellectual disability, some people with Down syndrome do *not* have an intellectual disorder; and 69% of people with autism do *not* have an intellectual disorder (Autism Speaks, 2022). That said, many research studies do not parse the different specific diagnoses within IDD, therefore, in this chapter we use the term IDD in a broad and inclusive way that characterizes a person who has deficits in cognitive, adaptive, mental, and/or other areas of functioning. Such cases would qualify for what *DSM-5* terms to be neurodevelopmental disorders (we cover other specific neurodevelopmental disorders in other chapters). In this chapter, when the scientific study has made diagnostic distinctions, we point those out, such as those that study intellectual disability *and* autism separately (e.g., Datu & Niemiec, 2023).

R. M. Niemiec, D. Tomasulo, *Character Strengths and Abilities Within Disabilities*, Positive Psychology and Disability Series,
https://doi.org/10.1007/978-3-031-36294-1_3

character strengths, positive emotional well-being, and growth (Albaum et al., 2021). That research highlights the importance of delving into character strengths science and practice for people with IDD. Building off the foundational concepts, research, and practices from the chapters in Part I, we delve into central ways character strengths integrate in helping educators, professionals, administrators, and other leaders think in new, expansive, and truly inclusive ways. These help to create a character strengths-mindset that aligns with a character strengths-based approach. To tailor the mindset and approach to IDD, we begin with seven core insights.

1. *Character strengths offer a language of inclusiveness*

If someone is including others or taking an organizational approach of inclusion, that person is using character strengths. At its core, inclusion involves fairness and justice in action toward others. Indeed, one cannot include others without tapping into character strengths. As we look more deeply we see that all the character strengths are present. Inclusion involves the strength of perspective—seeing the bigger picture of its importance. It takes the strength of leadership to incite the approach, bravery to challenge an antiquated system, and teamwork and perseverance to carry it out. Individuals can be creative in their approach to involve those who are isolated, love of learning to delve into new approaches, and the strength of hope to aspire toward an environment that is appreciated by all and uses everyone's strengths and talents. Each of the 24 character strengths can be activated as a pathway or a direct expression of inclusion.

2. *Character strengths focus on ability*

Many strength-based approaches begin with a reframe from disability to ability, to remind consumers, readers, participants, and constituents that the work to be engaged in will not begin from a one-down approach or a mindset of "dis" or "without." Rather, such approaches begin by focusing on abilities, capacities, and strengths of individuals and groups. Arguably, the best starting point is who the person is—their core identity, that which forms what's best in them and makes them most energized and engaged—that is, their character strengths. Other strengths categories such as talents, skills, and interests are also important to round off a focus on the abilities of people.

3. *Character strengths are an equalizer*

Categorical systems such as the DSM-5 and ICD-11 place people in either-or categories, typically resulting in "in" or "out"—one has the diagnosis or one does not have the diagnosis. Pastimes take a similar approach in which one is on the winning team or the losing team, one has won the championship or has lost it. These approaches are distinct from the dimensional approach to character strengths of gradations and situational specificity—a person expressing more or less of a given character strength and expressing that strength level in variance based on the situation they are in.

All persons have potential to express their internal capacities and the focus is not a siloed "who's best at kindness or forgiveness?" rather it is the universal approach of "how might you—whomever you are—express kindness or forgiveness in this situation?" This is not the case for all strengths categories, for example, for strengths of abilities and intelligences there are some people who are far more talented at playing the violin, at basketball, or at computing complex mathematical formulas.

4. *Character strengths are a balancer of extremes*

There are many ways people engage with people with disabilities. It is not uncommon for people to fall into extremes. Common approaches include ignoring, placating, and the over-the-top cheerleader (e.g., "wow, you did great opening that gift, that's incredible"; "you are so amazing at everything"). At the other extreme is a discounting approach that assumes the worst of the person, never considers inclusion, and views the person as less than, weak, incapable, or fatally flawed. This discounting approach may be outside of people's conscious awareness. A balanced approach sees the humanity in the other, looks for what is best, and can see the reality of strengths and weaknesses; in other words, seeing and connecting with the humanness of the person with a disability, as with others.

Another way to think about the role of character strengths as a balancer is to consider how character strengths can balance strengths that are underused or overused (Niemiec, 2019). A person with Down syndrome may overuse their humor continuing to laugh and repeat the same joke even though it might be annoying or hurtful to others. The person can be given feedback to use their strength of kindness to be caring to others in the situation, to see that their humor might be viewed as unkind, and that instead of telling the joke to think of a kind act to display instead. This approach to balancing an overused strength is known as the tempering effect (Niemiec, 2019). Another example is a person with autism who underuses their strength of gratitude as evidenced by never expressing thankfulness or any form of appreciation to a classmate who is regularly giving extra time and support to them. Upon observing this, a teacher, counselor, or support staff might point out the importance of gratitude and turn to the person with autism's signature strength to help. This is known as the tempering effect and is another way to bring balance to strengths (Niemiec, 2019). In this example, the person with autism is highest in love of learning and is encouraged to spend time learning about gratitude, its rationale and importance, and reading about examples of how to express it in action.

5. *A character strengths approach is a growth mindset approach*

To take on a growth mindset is to understand we can growth through hard work and dedication, as opposed to growing through talent or intelligence alone (Dweck, 2006). Growth mindset involves looking for opportunities at times of difficulty and learning at times of failure. While no person is always in a growth mindset, there are several characteristics that can help capture such a mindset in a given situation. Table 3.1 explains several elements of growth mindset alongside character strengths we suggest are at the core of each.

In addition to the alignment of character strengths with the core elements of growth mindset itself, any of the 24 character strengths can be the subject themselves for a growth mindset of learning and improving. Research on adolescents has

Table 3.1 Growth mindset elements and hypothesized character strengths components

Growth mindset tenet	Character strength rationale
Achievements are due, in large part, to effort (not just inherent talent)	*Perseverance* is the energy and effort to keep going despite hardship and challenges
Willingness to learn from mistakes and from criticism	*Love of learning* to deepen one's knowledge; *judgment/critical thinking* to appreciate alternative views
Intelligence and ability can be developed	*Hope* to expect the best and think toward possibilities, capacities, and development
Ask questions and admit when something is not known	*Curiosity* to inquire, search, and explore; *humility* to let go of the ego and the need to know everything
Seeking out challenging tasks and taking on risks	*Bravery* to face adversity and difficulties as needed

found that having a growth mindset about strengths is connected with greater well-being and strengths use (Jach et al., 2018).

Who takes a character strengths approach? Might it be certain people—professionals and non-professionals—who are high in certain character strengths? A large-scale study looked at stigmatization and found that the character strengths of kindness, fairness, and social intelligence were most linked to being less stigmatizing toward people with autism and people with IDD (Datu & Niemiec, 2023). Other very strong correlations were for leadership, love, and bravery. Self-regulation was associated with higher stigmatization for IDD and autism (also perseverance for autism only). While these findings do not point to a proven intervention around deploying certain character strengths to reduce stigma and enhance a character strengths-based, growth-oriented approach, they provide some foundation for immediate reflection and further study.

6. *Character strengths are critical for managing adversity*

Disability, by nature, brings forth unique challenges and stressors. Many people with IDD face additional physical, psychological, and social problems (Gilmore & Cuskelly, 2014; Wehmeyer, 2013). Theories in character strengths show character to be a critical—and often untapped—avenue for addressing adversity and cultivating resilience (Niemiec, 2020).

Adversity can come in other forms such as the ways that the environment or context (e.g., work, school, community) excludes, obstructs, or limits the person, such as access issues, transportation issues, policy issues, and social norms, to name a few. The environment has generally been shaped for people without disabilities and is therefore incompatible for a range of disabilities (Wehmeyer, 2013). If each environmental obstacle is called out and focused on individually, it can be faced with strengths of character. No adversity or environmental obstacle will be overcome without character strengths such as perseverance, creativity, bravery, zest, fairness, and so on.

7. *Character strengths (and signature strengths) offer a pathway for belonging*

Loneliness is a substantial problem for people with IDD. A representative sample in England found that people with disability are far more likely to experience loneliness than people without disability (Emerson et al., 2021). These researchers examined disability in a general way (not only IDD) by asking whether the person had a physical or mental health condition/illness for 12 months or more and that has a negative impact on carrying out day-to-day activities. They discovered disability was connected with low perceived social support, social isolation, and lower well-being. Gilmore and Cuskelly (2014), in looking only at IDD (children and adults), reviewed the available evidence and found that about half of people with IDD were chronically lonely, which is far more than the general population of around 15–30%. These researchers also observed that people with IDD are highly vulnerable to loneliness.

One targeted remedy for loneliness is to help people with IDD build further social and community involvement, support, and integration, and more specifically, to facilitate belonging. Belonging is a fundamental human need to form and maintain strong relationships (Baumeister & Leary, 1995). At a basic level, when a person enters a new setting/situation, there are central questions they ask themselves in terms of their belonging; and there are optimal strategies that can be taken to support individuals (Walton & Brady, 2017). Signature strengths, an individual's highest, most essential qualities of personality, are aligned conceptually with these strategies. Table 3.2 offers four of these common questions that run through people's mind when they enter a new setting and whether or not they belong or could

Table 3.2 Belonging questions, strategies, and signature strengths alignments

Questions on belonging (Walton & Brady, 2017)	Supportive strategy (Walton & Brady, 2017)	Signature strengths alignment with strategies
Does anyone here even notice me?	Recognize and acknowledge people	Naming or noticing a person's signature strength(s) in an interaction helps the person feel "seen" and appreciated (e.g., Niemiec, 2018)
Are there people here whom I connect with?	Build a sense of personal connection to others there	Sharing similar top strengths builds a feeling of intimacy and connection (Kashdan et al., 2018)
Do people here value/like me?	Provide a narrative to understand common challenges in the setting so as to not block one's belonging; broaden representation of who belongs	Explaining that all 24 character strengths matter and that whichever strengths a person is high in, that can be valued, important, and can make a contribution to the group (Niemiec & Pearce, 2021)
Is this a setting in which I want to belong?	Represent the setting as a way to offer opportunities to pursue valued goals	Explaining that signature strengths offer a pathway to reach personal or shared goals (e.g., Linley et al., 2010)

belong (Walton & Brady, 2017). Strategies and signature strengths alignment with each are included.

Belonging has also been studied with IDD populations. Erik Carter (2016; Carter et al., 2016) conducted in-depth interviews of people with IDD and their families, examining themes that reflected a trajectory of deepening relationships; the context of their focus was belonging in the faith congregational setting. They identified ten themes of belonging for people with IDD (which could be applied to people without IDD as well). These ten are: being present, invited, welcomed, known, accepted, supported, cared for, befriended, needed, and loved. These dimensions reflect deepening relationships and are reflective of an inclusive community. While character strengths have not been examined in terms of these belonging dimensions, there seems to be a strong alignment. We suggest the following connections:

1. Character strengths important to building positive relationships, such as love, kindness, and teamwork (Wagner et al., 2019) may align with facilitating belonging.
2. Character strengths important to building friendships, such as honesty, humor, kindness, and fairness (Wagner, 2018), may align with facilitating belonging.
3. The importance of recognizing and appreciating signature strengths (Kashdan et al., 2018)—as mentioned alongside the belonging questions and strategies—would likely be relevant to these belonging dimensions as well.

The Science

Approaches to intellectual/developmental disability has been traditionally entrenched in diagnostic-focused, medical models and deficit-based, psychological models geared toward psychopathology, inabilities, and/or the presence of "negative" emotions, constructs, and problems (Danforth, 2001; Dykens, 2006; Niemiec et al., 2017; Wehmeyer, 2013). The scientific literature mirrors such disability approaches for IDD. That said, the integration of strengths-based approaches for people with IDD has been slowly evolving and has been placing emphasis on the skills, resources, interests, and abilities of people with IDD. We refer to this important shift as Strengths-Based: Phase 1.

Researchers sounded a call to the disability field to take strengths-based approaches further—more systematically and scientifically-based—to highlight and build character strengths to assess, empower, treat, and care for people with IDD (Niemiec et al., 2017). We refer to this expansion of strengths to integrate who the person is at their core (i.e., their character strengths) as an evolution to Strengths-Based: Phase 2. This phase applies the latest science and best practices in an empowering way to individuals and groups. It has also been noted that working with character strengths in these ways for people with IDD is not only positive and likely beneficial to individuals, but is a low-cost approach (Raley et al., 2020).

We highlight several studies in character strengths and IDD, centered around the following four areas: assessment, staff character strengths, the character strengths of people with IDD, and outcomes.

Assessment Measures

A number of positive constructs have been examined in people with disabilities. For example, in a study of adolescents with and without cognitive disabilities, the constructs of hope, optimism, locus of control, and self-determination were measured and both hope and optimism predicted life satisfaction in the youth with and without disability (Shogren et al., 2006). There are a number of positive-oriented, well-being focused measures specific for IDD, such as the PHI-Intellectual Disabilities measure which is a short well-being assessment with good psychometrics based on a sample of 130 people with IDD (Monterde et al., 2022). There are also a number of short measures of well-being that could be adapted for people with IDD such as the five-item, Satisfaction with Life Scale (Diener et al., 1985). Indeed, entire textbooks have been written about positive psychological assessment (e.g., Ruch et al., 2022), and many of the measures could be adapted. The focus here, however, will be specific to the research on character strengths assessment for IDD.

An initial approach to character was developed prior to the VIA Classification work and is referred to as the Assessment Scale for Positive Character Traits-Developmental Disabilities (ASPeCT-DD) measure (Woodard, 2009). This is a valid measure of positive traits of people with IDD as observed by informants; the majority of traits measured are VIA character strengths, such as forgiveness, humor, gratitude, courage, self-control, kindness, and optimism/hope.

Following the advent of the VIA Classification in 2004, there emerged a growing need to assess character strengths in people with IDD. The formal study of the VIA Inventory of Strengths and its inclusiveness level for people with IDD began with researchers at Kansas University and the VIA Institute. The researchers compared youth with disabilities and youth without disabilities and found psychometric support for using the VIA Youth Survey with young people with IDD and other disabilities (Shogren et al., 2018). There were similarities in the reliability of scores across youth with and without disabilities, however, young people with disabilities tended to score lower on character strength than those without disabilities (Shogren et al., 2017a, b, 2018). This finding that younger people with disabilities tend to rate themselves lower on positive constructs has also been shown with self-determination measures; this issue points to the possible factor of the environment influencing beliefs of youth (Shogren et al., 2016).

Additional work on the language of the VIA measures has extended to adults with IDD by Schwartz et al. (2022). Their work on the 24 character strengths involves improving the measurement items to be more concrete without colloquialisms and symbolic terms. This work is ongoing but interviews with people with IDD have revealed the VIA assessment increases their self-knowledge and self-esteem. In addition, preliminary data reveal that the character strengths that were more challenging to understand were within the strengths of creativity, fairness, hope, and spirituality, while the items that were easiest to understand were in the strengths of humor, kindness, perseverance, and self-regulation (Schwartz, 2022). The more challenging items seemed to be due to the lack of concrete examples and thereby are more abstract in nature, while the strengths that were easier to understand seem to be aligned with the social narrative around disability such as the kind and funny person who should work hard (perseverance) and behave well and be in control (self-regulation) (Schwartz, 2022).

Character Strengths and Staff

Schwartz et al. (2022) studied clinicians using the VIA measures with adults with IDD and found a myriad of practical uses, including the fostering of self-understanding and self-esteem, providing a framework for understanding strengths, supporting communication across service systems, and the shaping of strengths-based interventions. In a different study of treatment program/school staff of people supporting clients with autism and other developmental disorders, the VIA Inventory was administered (Korn et al., 2016). The top strengths of staff were kindness, honesty, humor, fairness, and love. The researchers observed that these character strengths were contagious and had reciprocal benefit from staff to individuals. This appears to reflect a *virtuous circle* of mutual strengths expression that can occur between two or more people such as those working together, supervising/leading, or supporting others (Niemiec, 2014, 2018). When Korn and colleagues (2016) interviewed the staff and analyzed the benefits of using their character strengths with individuals with IDD, they discovered a host of powerful findings: character strengths helped them to motivate clients, to build their strengths, to maximize progress, to avoid negative outcomes, to promote coping, to build strong relationships, meet those with unique needs, and to do the "right" thing.

In a study of developmental services workers, the top character strengths were humor, teamwork, fairness, honesty, kindness, self-regulation, love of learning, and perspective. Interviews found that workers used character strengths to provide compassionate and meaningful care, motivate their own flourishing at work, and to support their clients' well-being (Darewych et al., 2020).

Character Strengths of Individuals

In a unique study comparing people with and without autism, it was found that while the strengths were similar, people with autism report less knowledge and use of their strengths; and when strengths use is reported in people with autism there is a higher quality of life, well-being, and mental health than those with autism using their strengths less frequently (Taylor et al., 2023). Another study of people with autism who completed the VIA Survey found that honesty, appreciation of beauty, love of learning, fairness, and kindness were the highest self-reported character strengths, while greater life satisfaction was associated with gratitude, hope, and honesty (Nocon et al., 2022).

In an international study of 306 people with IDD, including autism, the top five character strengths scores were love of learning, honesty, fairness, judgment, and appreciation of beauty. The bottom five character strengths scores were self-regulation, perseverance, zest, spirituality, and leadership (Umucu et al., 2022). These researchers observed that the ratings of strengths were lower among people with IDD than other disability groups and that therefore strength identification needs bolstering among people with IDD. This research with adults with IDD mirrors the research with adolescents mentioned earlier by Shogren and colleagues (2016, 2017a, b) in regard to lower character strengths ratings by people with IDD. Umucu et al. (2022) observed that those with IDD had love of learning endorsements higher than other disability groups, which reflects a strong desire to grow and learn new topics.

A national agency in the United States called START which offers direct services to people with developmental disabilities, embeds character strengths in their services. At intake, each client either receives the VIA Survey and completes it themselves or the staff engages in character strengths-spotting through the intake process and discussions to arrive at the client's top character strengths. In tracking a sampling of intake strengths-spotting (N = 3010) and formal VIA Survey takers (N = 188), the top five character strengths through these two very different processes were identical! While in different order for each, the top strengths identified were love, kindness, humor, curiosity, and creativity (Beasley et al., 2023). In addition, appreciation of beauty, love of learning, and honesty were in the top 10 for both assessment approaches, while bravery, perseverance, zest, hope, and gratitude rounded out as the identical top 13 strengths in each approach, showing remarkable reliability across two approaches measuring character strengths in large samples of people with IDD.

Parent reports of their children with autism has been a source for learning about strengths. Some studies have looked at both the parent and the individual's reports of character strengths. Kirchner et al. (2016) examined individuals with Asperger's Disorder and neurotypical controls and found that the former were highest in judgment/critical thinking, creativity, and love of learning (cognitive strengths) while the latter were highest in kindness, fairness, humor, love (social/emotional strengths). It was the social and emotional strengths that had the highest positive connections with life satisfaction for the Asperger's group. Samson and Antonelli (2013) focused in on the character strength of humor among people with Asperger's and found that it was the 16th highest strength on average compared with typically developing individuals (matched by age, gender, and education) in which humor ranked 8th. They also found that when examined alongside types of happiness (pleasurable/hedonic happiness and eudaimonic types of happiness such as engagement and meaning), for people with Asperger's, humor was related only to pleasure while for typically developing individuals humor was related to pleasure, engagement, and meaning.

A qualitative study of parent reports of their child (an adolescent or adult) with IDD or autism found that the most reported positive qualities were personality-related (82%) and sociability (53%) with most parents reporting one or more qualities (97%) (Wilkinson et al., 2022). In another study, the VIA Classification was used as a framework for coding 153 parents' descriptions of the best things about their children. With the ages ranging from 3 to 11, the most common, parent-endorsed strengths were love, kindness, and humor, across all ages, while the strength of perseverance was highly endorsed when the children entered school. Higher scores on the Child Behavior Checklist (a validated instrument used to detect behavioral/emotional problems) was connected with lower likelihood of endorsing humanity-oriented character strengths (Cost et al., 2021).

Looking to other family members' reports, Carter et al. (2020) examined how people with IDD and autism were perceived by their siblings. They found moderate to high ratings of character strengths by the siblings. The majority of individuals were described as having multiple character strengths, indicating not only the ease of identifying character strengths but the high degree of character strengths perceived in siblings with IDD.

The observations of the character strengths of students on the autism spectrum has also been studied in teachers/educators. Across ages 7–8 and 10–11, kindness, self-regulation, and perseverance were the strengths most endorsed, while there was a decreased endorsement of courage strengths when the student scored high in challenging behavior or symptoms severity (Mirenda et al., 2022).

Character Strengths Outcomes

The science on character strengths outcomes with people with IDD is slowly emerging, both inside and outside the education context. Linkins et al. (2014) offered several strategies for applying character strength in the education context involving four major areas including, developing a character strengths language and lens using the VIA Survey; recognizing and thinking about character strengths in others and in oneself; practicing with and applying character strengths; and identifying, celebrating, and cultivating group character strengths. These areas were applied and tested in an integrated classroom in Europe with children with and without disabilities to reduce discrimination between children and improve class climate (Bressoud et al., 2018). Feedback revealed that this application was feasible for IDD and advocated for wider application to other classrooms, schools, and even the entire system of education. Coppley and Niemiec (2021) outline several examples and cases involving applying character strengths in public education systems, where approximately 15% of students have disabilities that receive support (Institute of Education Sciences, 2022).

Multi-week intervention programs with character strengths have been conducted. For example, one controlled intervention study examined neurodivergent children in early childhood education. The intervention involved eight 30-min interventions in the classroom focusing on multiple specific character strengths (i.e., gratitude, optimism/hope, perseverance, and zest) and showed initial benefits such as for teacher-rated executive functioning (Naples & Tuckwiller, 2021). A 16-week intervention study in Europe, among fourth through sixth graders, focused on teaching children character strengths awareness and use to promote learning, well-being, and social skills. Benefits included consistency of interest, group cohesion, and classroom spirit. Examples of benefits revealed in teacher interviews included naming strengths in others, support for one another, well-being, and positive interactions (Vuorinen et al., 2018).

There is exciting research on belonging and IDD, an area mentioned earlier in the chapter that holds substantial potential. Carter and colleagues (2015) found that higher ratings of character strengths were predicted by greater involvement in community activities and that challenging behaviors predicted lower ratings of strengths (Carter et al., 2015). These findings point to the importance of emphasizing inclusion and connection in the community as well as fostering opportunities for people with IDD to be present and to feel invited, welcomed, known, accepted, supported, cared for, befriended, needed, and loved (Carter, 2016).

Among many findings in a study of well-being among 389 youth with autism and/or intellectual disability, higher well-being ratings in one or more domains was predicted by youth character strengths, as well as faith, community involvement, and minority status (Biggs & Carter, 2015). Another well-being study found that across two studies, hope was the character strength most linked with life satisfaction for people with Asperger's (Kirchner et al., 2016).

As the research in character strengths for people with IDD continues to gain blossom, these aforementioned studies lay an important foundation for the science, pointing toward not only positive benefits but new horizons.

The Practice

As indicated in the previous section, studies have shown that practices with character strengths are not only feasible to implement but can be successful for people with IDD. In this section, we delve into a range of practical assessment and intervention strategies.

Assessment as Intervention

An important first step in the practice of character strengths is assessment; this means to find a pathway—the more research-validated the better—to measure character strengths in the individual or group. Practitioners and scientists are reminded here that assessment is an intervention itself, and is personal and substantive, especially when measuring positive qualities that typically go unnoticed and unexplored.

We suggest that there are several levels by which character strengths can be measured that can be tailored to the individual with IDD. We begin with the standard, validated approach and progress toward different adaptations:

1. The individual takes the online VIA Inventory of Strengths (colloquially known as the VIA Survey; for ages 18 and up) or the VIA Inventory of Strengths for Youth (colloquially known as the VIA Youth Survey; for ages 8–17). They take the test on their own, with no support. These are the gold-standard, validated measures of character strengths, with a large number of validated translations to other languages. The former is 96 questions (four questions per strength) and the latter is 98 questions (four questions per strength with the exception of teamwork which is six questions). If the individual takes the VIA Inventory, they are part of a global response of 30 million survey takers (as of mid-2023).
2. The individual takes either VIA instrument with the support of someone, such as a parent, professional, or employer, using a central support document. Shogren et al. (2015) created a document to be used by people supporting youth with varying levels of IDD to help them take a VIA measure in an ideal way that adheres to general test parameters and avoids too much adult influence. The document contains general and item-specific recommendations, accommodations, cognitive supports, rewording strategies, and examples.
3. Administer a shorter validated measure of character strengths such as the "Signature Strengths Survey" or the "Global Assessment of Character Strengths." Although these are different types of measurement tools, these accomplish the intention of measuring top strengths and offer brevity.
4. Offer a list of the 24 character strengths with abbreviated, concrete definitions. The individual themselves or with a support person goes through the words and meanings and circles those strengths that "best describe who they are." The first two columns of Table 3.3 offer this approach.
5. Arrange for the individual's network (e.g., family members, professionals, peers, co-workers) to complete a Character Strengths 360 on the individual's behalf. This is a popular exercise used around the world across populations and has been found to elicit unique insights, stories, and strengths data about the person (found in Niemiec, 2014, 2018). A variation of this approach would be to distribute what is discussed in #4 to the person's network. After several people complete the measure on the individual's behalf, the data are compiled, summarized, and examined for top strengths discovered across people or across contexts.
6. The individual's parent, guardian, or support professional who knows them well completes the VIA Survey or VIA Youth Survey on the individual's behalf. This approach might be used for those with certain communication or comprehension challenges. This approach can yield helpful information for those who work with and care for the individual.

Each of these assessment approaches is free, as are the 20 validated character strengths measures found at VIA Institute on Character (2022). That site also

Table 3.3 Character strengths with user-friendly descriptions, examples, and action steps

Character strength	Description	Example	Practical action to take
Creativity	You like to create unique things that are of use. You can think of many different ways to solve a problem	A young man who plays the guitar for his class each week decides to wear a unique outfit for each show	Do an activity in a new way. Create something new (art, music, writing)
Curiosity	You like to explore things. You are very interested in trying out new activities and meeting new people	A young child asks her parents several questions about each city while on vacation	Ask a friend something you have never asked them. Explore a new topic
Judgment	You are logical and like to think. When someone gives an opinion you like to examine it in many different ways	A teen tries different approaches to program a TV remote, thinking about all his options	Look at the details of a situation. Be open to other ideas
Love of learning	You want to keep learning. You love to deepen your knowledge. You spend a lot of time learning as much as you can	An adult has an interest in learning a lot on a particular topic and takes college classes	Learn one new thing in every situation
Perspective	You are wise. You learn from your mistakes. You offer guidance to others who are struggling	A friend is upset after his basketball team loses. His friend tells him: "It's OK. It's only a game"	Offer advice to a friend who needs help
Bravery	You face your fears. When there is a problem, you go right toward it to solve it. You stand up for what is right	A young woman is nervous about public speaking. She takes a deep breath, faces her fear, and steps up to the stage	Face what you are afraid of. Challenge yourself
Perseverance	When you have a goal, you keep going. You overcome anything that might get in your way. You finish what you start	A young adult repeats her personal motto to herself when she is stressed: "Just do it. I will do my best"	Don't give up when something is difficult. Keep trying
Honesty	You tell the truth. You are viewed by others as sincere and genuine	A little girl exclaims that even though it's not always comfortable, she chooses to tell the truth to people	Tell people the truth. Be "the real you"
Zest	You are full of energy. You are enthusiastic about life. You always seem to be talking to people	A friendly adolescent is always the first to greet people at each activity and sporting event	Take action! Move your body!
Love	You are loving toward others and you receive love from others. You value being close to people	An adolescent hugs others in a warm, caring way following a positive interaction	Be a warm and strong listener; be genuine

(continued)

Table 3.3 (continued)

Character strength	Description	Example	Practical action to take
Kindness	You often do good things for people. You are helpful and caring. You are generous	A woman explains she gets great pleasure from being nice to people any time she can	Be nice and friendly. Be caring. Give your time to help others
Social intelligence	You are closely aware of your feelings and the feelings of others. You seem to say the right thing in many situations	A man noticed a sad expression on his co-worker's face and asked her how she was doing	Ask someone how they feel. Tell people how you feel
Teamwork	You value being a team player. You are loyal to your group. You always fulfill your duty on teams and in groups	A young woman decides to give back to her community by volunteering	Work side-by-side with 1 or more people. Spend time with groups
Fairness	You believe strongly in equality for everyone. You treat people the way you want to be treated.	A woman demands justice to her supervisor when she sees a co-worker being mistreated	Treat someone the way you want to be treated
Leadership	You are good at organizing groups of people. You would much rather be the leader than a follower in a group	A man explains he enjoys being an advocate for people who do not have "a voice"	Organize an activity for a group. Share an idea for the group to do
Forgiveness	You often give people a second chance after they have harmed you. You are good at letting things go	In response to being teased, a man decides to simply walk away and "let it go"	Let a hurt feeling go. Accept someone's weakness
Humility	You are a modest person. You do not brag about yourself. You place the attention on other people	A musician shares how he is happy to perform on stage but to let others get the attention	Let others talk about their success. Don't brag when you do well
Prudence	You are cautious to not take too many risks. You are good at planning. You are responsible and usually on time	An adult is described by friends as very organized and committed to his goals	Think first! Pause before you take a risk. Be careful
Self-regulation	You are disciplined. You are good at handling stress. You control your bad habits (e.g., eating, drinking)	A woman announces to her family that she has decided to quit smoking	Take control of your anger. Take care of yourself
Appreciation of beauty	You often observe beauty around you. You are filled with wonder. You want what you and others do to be "just right"	A man walks into a museum and marvels at the beauty and precision of the artwork	Find beauty in nature, art, ideas, and when people are good

(continued)

Table 3.3 (continued)

Character strength	Description	Example	Practical action to take
Gratitude	You often feel grateful for your life and for the good things that happen. You almost always tell people "thank you"	A couple expresses their appreciation for having connected with a new friend	Tell people "thank you." Explain why you are grateful
Hope	You are optimistic. You are positive. You often look to the future and see good things	A young woman describes the optimism of her roommate: "She looks forward, and only forward"	Be positive, especially when others are not. Look for the good in people
Humor	You love to make people smile and laugh. You are playful with people. You turn gloomy situations into fun ones	A man is playful and mischievous with his group; he makes others smile and laugh with each joke	Smile! Tell jokes. Laugh a lot, *with* others
Spirituality	You are filled with a sense of life purpose and meaning. You practice a particular faith or set of beliefs	A young man takes walks in nature to be in touch with the animals, trees, and "life" all around him	What matters most to you? Do that. Find your purpose

enables free data collection of groups of students, employees, clients, or research subjects using any of the measures and is used by hundreds of researchers every year.

Initial Action Steps

After participants have taken a character strengths assessment, they are often eager to put their new learnings into action. Many practitioners and educators deploying character strengths interventions with people with IDD remark that the most important strategy or resource needed is user-friendly, practical suggestions for each of the 24 strengths. In addition to plain language definition and examples, Table 3.3 offers one practical suggestion that could be used as a next step for each character strength, with the intention of accessibility for people with IDD. These can be considered starting points for conversations, brainstorming, and even for a daily practice to boost the strength.

To extend the practical applications for IDD, we turn to Niemiec et al. (2017) who, in their flagship article on character strengths for the IDD field, compiled an array of positive psychology interventions based on the literature at that time. Their emphasis was on interventions that might be most easily adapted for IDD populations, such as building the skill of spotting character strengths. Among the activities, there were strategies that focused on specific character strength such as kindness or gratitude and there were strategies that could be individualized to any person, such

Table 3.4 Character strengths interventions that can be used and adapted for people with IDD

Intervention	Explanation	Scientific base
Use a signature strength	Identify one of your highest 5 strengths and use it in a new way each day	Schutte and Malouf (2019)
Build the skill of strengths-spotting in others	Look for the strengths of others in action; spot and explain what is observed	Quinlan et al. (2019)
Build the skill of strengths-spotting in yourself	Examine stories of when one was at one's best, highly engaged, or particularly happy. Make note of the character strengths in each story and how they were used	Seligman et al. (2005)
Character strengths 360	Gather feedback about one's top 5 strengths and examples from several people in different contexts in one's life; examine patterns	Niemiec (2018)
Acting "as if"	Name the character strength one wants to improve and the situation where it could be used. Act in a way that is consistent with that strength in that situation	Blackie et al. (2014)
Set goals with aware-explore-apply	Name the strength one wants to become more aware of. Explore examples of past use of the strength. Set an action plan to apply the strength	Niemiec (2014)
Target a happiness strength (zest)	Increase one's activity each day through walking/ movement, exercising, or other activities	Proyer et al. (2013)
Target a happiness strength (hope)	Visualize and write about one's best possible self at a future timepoint. See the details in a realistic, positive way. Consider the character strengths pathways that will be needed	Meevissen et al. (2011)
Target a happiness strength (curiosity)	Select a task that you do each week that you don't like (e.g., washing dishes, vacuuming). Pay attention (be curious) about three novel features about the activity, using the senses	Langer (2006)
Count kindness	Track the kind actions one takes for 1 week	Otake et al. (2006)
Count blessings	Write down 3 things one is grateful for each day and why they occurred	Gander et al. (2013)
Name 3 funny things	Write down 3 things that were funny each day and what made them funny	Wellenzohn et al. (2016)

as using a signature strength in a new way. We expand upon this list to offer additional character strengths activities with an evidence base that can be adapted for people with IDD. Table 3.4 includes activities from Niemiec et al. (2017) and the additional interventions, many of which are described in Niemiec (2018); it also offers an explanation of the activity, and the evidence base (limited to one citation for each). Every individual with IDD is unique so the adaptations should not be viewed as universal for all, rather they are meant as an additional lens to be considered. The first six entries are general strategies that can be tailored to any character strength while the latter six target specific strengths.

Strengths-Spotting

Strengths-spotting means to *spot*, *explain*, and *appreciate* the character strengths in oneself or others (the SEA model, Niemiec, 2018). This involves "seeing" the person by their core qualities, giving behavioral evidence for what is seen, and affirming or giving value to the person for those best qualities. We have taught this approach to tens of thousands of people across the globe and while the positive impact is often immediate, the impact for people with IDD is especially powerful. As opposed to a focus on deficits, areas they need to improve upon, or generic things they like to do, the focal point is that which is most central to them as a human being, how that is uniquely expressed, and how it can bring benefit to them. Consider the following two real world examples of different medical specialists meeting a 2-year-old young child with an IDD for an initial visit.

The specialist came into the exam room. She did not greet the parents but began the conversation immediately.

"So, he failed his 2 tests last week," the doctor said.

"Well, actually," the father said, "two people that read the tests last week said that he was in the moderate range for one test and for the other test he was slightly under the level he needed to be."

"No, he failed them both," the doctor responded.

End of conversation.

On an initial visit, the same child was seen by a different specialist.

The doctor walked in the room, greeted the parents and then paused to look at the young boy. The boy moved his legs and arms quickly up and down and swayed his body from side to side.

"Wow, he is vigorous. What great energy he is showing!" she exclaimed.

She continued to observe and examine the boy.

"I can tell he is hardworking. Despite his bronchiolitis, he is putting forth good effort with his breathing. He just keeps trying and trying. He's not giving up."

The parents and physician discussed the treatment of bronchiolitis while the physician watched the child out of the corner of her eye.

"And I also want to point out how inquisitive he is. He keeps looking over to where we are and each time a toy or something is placed in front of him, he wants to explore that toy."

It is likely that neither of these two physicians had any formal training in the science of positive psychology or character strengths. However, the second physician was naturally oriented toward the skill of strengths-spotting, as she easily spotted and verbalized the child's strengths with the words "vigorous" (i.e., zest), "hardworking" (i.e., perseverance), and "inquisitive" (curiosity). The impact on the observing parents was an immediate shot of well-being, greater engagement with the physician, and deeper appreciation of their child. While seeming to be simple, casual, and in-the-moment, strengths-spotting can sometimes seem to be a herculean task when one considers the deficit-focused medical culture, the professional demands (and rewards) to diagnosing and spotting flaws, the busyness of medical practice, and the hardwiring of all humans to notice what is wrong. At the same time, the approach of seeing people through the lens of strengths and weaving strengths into the existing conversation can be embedded by anyone and with someone at any age of life.

In some cases, strengths-spotting may require a gentle push by the caregiver, advocate, or professional. An example of this can be seen when I (RMN) went to pick up one of my children (who has Down syndrome) from daycare. I would ask the daycare workers how the day was for them. One particular daycare worker would see me and immediately announce her observations of my son—all negative and the majority trivial (e.g., he did not come the first time he was called for lunch, or he took another child's toy during the chaotic free play period). After several days of this pattern, I asked the worker my standard question about how the day went and again she offered her standard approach. I then said, "OK, thank you for sharing that. We will work on that. And, what did you notice that went right for him today? What was best about his day?" She was surprised at this question, thought for a moment, and offered two positive behaviors my son displayed during the day (i.e., at lunch he ate all his meal; at free play, he engaged in parallel play with two peers). I thank her for the observation. However, what was more remarkable was that simple (extra) question caused a shift in her. From that point forward, day after day, she shared positive observations in her report (although not neglecting his areas of struggle). I noticed that each day forward she was eager to share the positives with me (sometimes seeking me out to do so!) and it was clear she had given some attention to look for the good during the day.

Another example comes from one of our practitioner colleagues, Katie Curran, who shared her approach with people with autism which reflects the many ways she uses character strengths identification, spotting, and exploration. As an intervention she leads with adolescents, she embeds a variety of strengths-spotting strategies (Curran, personal communication, 2022). Here are some of the open-ended and closed-ended questions she offers conversationally with dyads/pairs:

- Who is high in the fairness strength? And who has leadership as a top strength?
- What does the strength of creativity mean? How have you used it?
- (Asking one teen about the other) How does Bobby use his honesty strength?
- (Asking one teen about the other) What is a character strength you see in Jake?
- (Asking one teen about the other) What do you like about Bobby's strength of bravery?

The layers of the SEA model are embedded in these questions and within the overall approach. The different framing for each question allows for a myriad of ways for others to learn about character strengths—in oneself, in others, and as qualities to explore and appreciate.

Another example of character strengths-spotting comes from the group context. In leading multiple strengths-spotting groups for people with IDD, we have found the following agenda and steps to be successful for a one-hour group experience.

This agenda assumes each participant's highest two (or more) character strengths have been identified prior to the group experience:

- Introduction: character strengths are explained as one's best qualities that can be developed and spotted in others.
- Sharing signature strengths: each individual shares their top two signature strengths and is prompted to give at least one example of how they have used one of the strengths.
- Spontaneous strengths-spotting: after a participant shares, the group is prompted with the question, "Are there any other character strengths you can spot in Zack?"
- The facilitator may need to support some participants in the strengths identification, and if one participant does not have strengths spontaneously spotted by the group on their turn (although this is quite rare amidst a group that is verbal), the facilitator is ready to point out strengths in that individual.
- Summary: facilitator reiterates the value of strengths-spotting, offers group highlights, and encourages participants to practice strengths-spotting each day with people in their life.

Our observations in these groups, albeit anecdotal evidence, reveals several insights including:

- All character strengths can be spotted in oneself and in others with IDD.
- Participants can connect strengths to behaviors and stories in their own lives.
- Participants are highly enthusiastic about spotting the character strengths of their peers.
- Participants experience joy, energy, and confidence in being part of such a group.

In our tracking of the character strengths observed, we found that the most frequent strengths spotted and discussed during these group activities were creativity, bravery, honesty, love, humor, love of learning, teamwork, forgiveness, and kindness. The least spotted and discussed strengths were prudence, social intelligence, perspective, judgment/critical thinking, and self-regulation. The least common strengths might require some additional explanation and concrete examples to support their identification and discussion. That said, two of these strengths (self-regulation and prudence) are consistently among the least common strengths on the VIA Inventory of Strengths across the globe (McGrath, 2015). It is interesting to compare these self-identifications/self-endorsements of character strengths (likened to an approach of "that's me") in comparison with the data discussed earlier around character strengths that may be least comprehended using a measurement approach (Schwartz et al., 2022).

Case Example: The Uncomfortable Friend

Research by Scope investigated perceptions of people with disabilities and found that 2/3 of people felt uncomfortable talking to a person with a disability (Aiden & McCarthy, 2014). This study in England also found that the discomfort is often due to a concern with saying the wrong thing or being patronizing, and ultimately a lack of experience with people with disabilities. Character strengths offer an important opportunity to have an impact, as evidenced in the following scenario.

Two adolescent friends, Jayden and Thomas, played sports outside with one another each day in the hot summer sun. On several occasions, they went inside to cool off and play video games in Thomas' house. Thomas' brother, Pete, who has an IDD, would often join them. Pete was friendly and eager to play with his peers. Then, 1 day, at Jayden's family dinner table, Jayden shared with his parents that he was uncomfortable with Pete:

"I don't know what to say to him," Jayden remarked.

"Why can't you just treat him like any other friend, like you do with any kid in your class at school?" his mother wondered.

"It's different. I don't understand what he's saying some of the time. Then I'm uncomfortable not knowing what to say back. I make up stuff or I just say, "Yeah" or "OK, cool" and then I move on.

"Yes, on one hand it might seem different to interact with Pete," his mother agreed, "but isn't there some uncertainty with any new person you interact with? There is always some unknown. The other day you spoke about having difficulty talking with that girl you like in school."

"That's true."

"Have you considered what Pete's character strengths are?" his mother inquired further.

"His what?"

"Pete's strengths of character—his best qualities. You know, like creativity, curiosity, perseverance, and honesty."

"Right, I remember those," Jayden recalled from his learning the previous school year. "Well, let's see...Pete is fair as he's very good at taking turns with the video games we play. And, he always comes right up to me to talk to me so I would say that's pretty brave. I mean, if I did that, I would consider myself brave. He does ask me questions about what I like and about the games we are playing. I would consider that pretty curious."

"Those seem like some important qualities in Pete. Nice job in identifying them," observed Jayden's mother. "Perhaps you might think of Pete in those ways when you are playing together?"

Jayden followed through on this. He thought about Pete's fairness, bravery, and curiosity right before walking in Pete's and Thomas' house. When they played together, he observed those strengths in Pete and was on the lookout for other strengths. Jayden's new mindset washed away his discomfort. He and Pete became closer friends over the years.

This scenario represents both a common situation people with disabilities face (people feeling discomfort around them) and a concrete strategy for overcoming discomfort. Character strengths offer something tangible and meaningful to transform not only perceptions of the person with a disability but the conversation and interaction itself.

Intervention Adaptations

Depending on the severity level of the individual, there are a myriad of adaptations that can be deployed to support someone with IDD. It goes beyond the scope of this chapter to discuss all of this literature and these practices, however, we offer some examples that have been discussed in the character strengths context.

There are a number of programs and educational tools that were not originally created for people with IDD but if wisely and carefully adapted, could be of substantial benefit for a wider range of people. One example in the character strengths field is the evidenced-based program, mindfulness-based strengths practice (MBSP) (Niemiec, 2014), which has been shown to be superior across several variables in three published studies to the most popular mindfulness program across the globe, and systematic reviews of the program have pointed to several well-being benefits (Prasath et al., 2021). Shogren and colleagues (2017a) highlight the potential of adapting this program for people with IDD. As a result, an adaptation of MBSP for people with IDD has been drafted and initially tested; it is referred to as MBSP-Access (Niemiec et al., 2022). This program involves several layers of adaptation. There's a layer of content adaptation, in this case, taking each of the eight themes of MBSP—and the strengths activities and meditations—and creating a more concrete, simplified version. A second layer involves the integration of new research on mindfulness or strengths activities found beneficial for people with IDD, such as the soles of the feet meditation (Singh et al., 2003). Another layer involves integrating the evidence-based processes that underpin the optimal practitioner approach for supporting people with IDD, including the teaching style (e.g., offering a person-centered approach), the material itself (e.g., using visual teaching methods), and the method of teaching (e.g., repeating/practicing content, not stacking content).

Adaptations of group therapy (Yalom, 1995) have been successfully done for people with IDD. Interactive-behavioral therapy (IBT) integrates tenets of group therapy and psychodrama with positive psychology components such as character strengths (Tomasulo, 2014). Another adaptation is the integration of acting methods and creative dramatics with character strengths application as an effective treatment for people with intellectual and psychiatric disabilities (Tomasulo & Szucs, 2015). There are many additional ways that practitioners can be creative in engaging clients, students, or colleagues with IDD. For examples, researchers have used video feedback to creatively help people with IDD, especially those with little to no literacy, to explore and understand their character strengths (Szucs et al., 2019).

Individualized Plans

For this practical strategy, we outline two kinds of plans for people with IDD, both centered in the school context, however, the concepts can apply to other contexts such as planning and goal-setting at work and home. The two types of plans are the traditional Individualized Education Plans (IEP) and a plan we are introducing referred to as the Individualized Strengths Plan (ISP). To see a 1-page handout used to describe these two plans, see Appendix B.

IEP

Individualized Education Plans (IEPs) are required by law for every student in special education in public schools in the United States and similarly in many other countries. The language in the IEP explains that the plan must leverage the student's strengths, however, this has not been clearly defined and can be easily glossed over or placated in the plan. The common approach in schools is to interpret "strengths" as skills and therefore the student's functional skills (e.g., daily activity skills, mobility skills, safety skills, behavior skills, communication skills) or academic skills (e.g., learns new words quickly, knows many facts, or understands math skills) are emphasized. We offer discussion for bringing character strengths into the plans.

IEPs set the educational focus for people with IDD and IEP meetings commonly include teachers, physical/speech/occupational therapists, paraprofessionals, principals, case managers, parents, and, ideally, the individual/student themselves. However, many of these meetings do not involve the student despite it being potentially one of the most important discussions of the person's life. As mentioned, strengths can be quickly passed over to emphasize the student's academic and social struggles and weaknesses and the goals to remedy those struggles and weaknesses.

The integration of character strengths can be done in many ways at the meeting and in the goals and planning. Character strengths can be the goal itself (e.g., I will build up my bravery in social situations in the classroom) or the pathway to reach the goal (e.g., I will use my curiosity each time I am challenged by a math problem) (Niemiec, 2018).

To improve and truly adhere to a shift from deficit-based to character strengths-based, here are a few suggestions:

1. Include/invite students to all IEP meetings, if appropriate.
2. Start meetings by naming the student's *signature* strengths of character. Offer examples and stories of how the student has used these strengths at school (and home).
3. During the meeting, give space for the student to share, to offer feedback and ideas, to respond to reports, and to ask/answer questions.
4. Set goals that callout the use and development of the student's signature strengths at school.
5. For academic and/or social goals in the IEP, list at least one way the student can use one of their character strengths to reach the goal.

ISP

An Individualized Strengths Plan (ISP) is a plan—for people with or without IDD—that focuses on the student's strengths of character (other strength categories can be integrated). This concept originally came from discussions one of the authors (RMN) had with Neal Mayerson, the chairman of the VIA Institute and brother of Arlene Mayerson, one of the legal architects of the Americans with Disabilities Act of 1990. The ISP is a new approach that is being scientifically investigated. The structure and guiding questions/areas to complete are described below, and further general details can be found in Appendix B.

In an ISP, the focus can be on any strengths of the student and the ways to amplify, explore, reinforce, and collaborate with these strengths. The student's signature strengths are likely to be of highest importance in an ISP. A potential planning form might involve the following details:

- Identifying information
- Top 5 Signature strengths
- Personal goal (academic, social):
  - Complete this sentence: I want to be able to…
  - How I will use one or more of my signature strengths to reach my goal…
  - The activities I will practice to help me reach my goal…
  - What obstacles may arise?
  - I will know I have reached my goal when…
- Character strengths goal:
  - What is one character strength I would like to see grow?
  - Here are some ways I will explore or practice my strength…
  - What obstacles may arise?
  - I will know I have reached my goal when…
- Support from parent/guardian/others in the home environment

The process for the ISP is the student takes the VIA Youth Survey (or similar method as discussed earlier in this chapter). They meet with a support person (teacher, intervention specialist, coordinator) one-one-one to discuss their results and complete the ISP. This may take one or two meetings. The student brings the form to their parent/guardian at home for support, acknowledgement, and comments. This important step fosters greater school-home coordination as well as opens the possibilities for home support and goal integration. The student then begins to work on their two goals (both the personal goal with signature strengths embedded and the character strengths goal).

Then, short follow-up meetings are scheduled on a regular basis (e.g., weekly or biweekly) to check on progress and offer support. A reflection sheet can be implemented in these meetings. This is meant to be straightforward and concise. It includes:

- A place to check off each day that the goal was focused on
- One thing I did to help achieve my personal goal this week is…
- One thing I did to practice my character strength goal this week is…

Without deliberate character strengths planning, professionals, teachers, and administrations cannot expect students to wield and enhance their best qualities on their own. As Benjamin Franklin once said, "By failing to prepare, we are preparing to fail." By implementing ISPs and character strengths–infused IEPs, students are learning essential skills to use and value their best qualities, encourage the best qualities of their peers, and deploy those best qualities to help them soar toward their academic and social goals. In other words, they are doing what the adults in their life should also be doing - that is, weaving character strengths into everyday living.

Future Directions

There remains more we do not know than do know in terms of the integration of character strengths with people with IDD, therefore, a myriad of possibilities are available for scientists.

We begin by highlighting the need for further intervention studies focusing on the enhancement of well-being and resilience for people with IDD. Early studies have shown the positive role of specific strengths such as gratitude or working with signature strengths. Implementing, deepening, and adapting such interventions for people with IDD could bring a wide range of benefit to the individuals, helping professionals, and systems. Those benefits remain unexplored such as the ways in which character strengths foster positive relationships, nuances in developing achievement, and contributing to positive cultures and environments.

There are opportunities to take existing evidence-based programs and adapt them for people with IDD. The MBSP (mindfulness-based strengths practice) program discussed earlier is one example. In addition, there are programs created for people with IDD that do not explicitly involve character strengths and such additions would potentially be a value-add. Examples include positive behavior supports interventions, self-determination interventions, and many of the existing transition planning programs.

Key Takeaways

- Any professional supporting a person with an IDD can develop a character strengths mindset, which includes understanding that character strengths offer a language of inclusiveness, a growth mindset approach, a pathway for belonging, and help to foster well-being and resilience.
- The VIA Inventory of Strengths (VIA Survey) offers a validated, inclusive approach to measuring character strengths and there are at least six methods for adapting and delivering it to individuals and groups.

- Repeated studies have shown a range of character strengths can be high in people with IDD and that character strengths are easily observed and appreciated by parents and siblings.
- There are practical next steps a person with IDD can immediately take after completing the VIA Survey or VIA Youth Survey.
- There are several evidenced-based interventions suggested in the literature to help people with IDD gain benefits through their character strengths or their top signature strengths.
- The practice of strengths-spotting—seeing, explaining, appreciating character strengths (SEA model)—can be used by any professional, family member, or the individual themselves.
- Character strengths can be readily used to overcome the discomfort that arises for many people when speaking with someone with IDD.
- Character strengths–infused IEPs and ISPs (individualized strength plans) can be deployed by professionals and systems to take a more inclusive, holistic, accurate, and inspiring approach in helping people with IDD to thrive.
- Additional interventions with character strengths could be deployed for supporting professionals—to understand their own character strengths, learn ways to optimally deploy them for each unique individual with IDD, and to support them in procedural strategies such as in leading and debriefing character strengths-driven IEPs and ISPs.

References

Aiden, H. S., & McCarthy, A. (2014). *Current attitudes towards disabled people*. Scope. Available at: https://research-information.bris.ac.uk/ws/portalfiles/portal/88783477/Aiden_and_McCarthy_2014.pdf

Albaum, C., Chan, V., Sellitto, T., Vashi, N., Hastings, R. P., & Weiss, J. A. (2021). Redressing the balance: A systematic review of positive psychology in the intellectual disability literature. *International Review of Research in MR*. https://doi.org/10.1016/bs.irrdd.2021.08.003

Autism Speaks. (2022). *Autism statistics and facts*. Found at: https://www.autismspeaks.org/

Baumeister, R. F., & Leary, M. R. (1995). The need to belong: Desire for interpersonal attachments as a fundamental human motivation. *Psychological Bulletin, 117*(3), 497–529.

Beasley, J. B., Caoili, A., & Klein, A. (2023). The assessment of character strengths in people with developmental disabilities: Unpublished data. National Center for START Services, Institute on Disability.

Biggs, E. E., & Carter, E. W. (2015). Quality of life for transition-age youth with autism or intellectual disability. *Journal of Autism and Developmental Disorders*. https://doi.org/10.1007/s10803-015-2563-x

Blackie, L. E. R., Roepke, A. M., Forgeard, M. J. C., Jayawickreme, E., & Fleeson, W. (2014). Act well to be well: The promise of changing personality states to promote Well-being. In A. C. Parks & S. Schueller (Eds.), *The Wiley-Blackwell handbook of positive psychological interventions* (pp. 462–474). Wiley-Blackwell.

Bressoud, N., Shankland, R., Ruch, W., & Gay, P. (2018). *Character strengths and children with special needs: A way to promote well-being all together*. Conference paper: International Conference on Well-Being in Education Systems.

Carter, E. W. (2016). A place of belonging: Research at the intersection of faith and disability. *Review and Expositor, 113*(2), 167–180.

Carter, E. W., Boehm, T. L., Biggs, E. E., Annandale, N. H., Taylor, C. E., Loock, A. K., & Liu, R. Y. (2015). Known for my strengths: Positive traits of transition-age youth with intellectual disability and/or autism. *Research and Practice for Persons with Severe Disabilities, 40*(2), 101–119. https://doi.org/10.1177/1540796915592158

Carter, E. W., Biggs, E. E., & Boehm, T. L. (2016). Being present versus having a presence: Dimensions of belonging for young people with disabilities and their families. *Christian Education Journal, 13*(1), 127–146.

Carter, E. W., Carlton, M. E., & Travers, H. E. (2020). Seeing strengths: Young adults and their siblings with autism or intellectual disability. *Journal of Applied Research in Intellectual Disabilities*. https://doi.org/10.1111/jar.12701

Coppley, J., & Niemiec, R. M. (2021). Character strengths interventions, systems change, and positive education. In M. Kern & M. L. Wehmeyer (Eds.), *The Palgrave handbook on positive education*. Palgrave Macmillan.

Cost, K. T., Zaidman Zait, A., Mirenda, P., Duku, E., Zwaigenbaum, L., Smith, I. M., Ungar, W. J., Kerns, C., Bennett, T., Szatmari, P., Georgiades, S., Waddell, C., Elsabbagh, M., & Vaillancourt, T. (2021). "Best things": Parents describe their children with autism spectrum disorder over time. *Journal of Autism and Developmental Disorders*. https://doi.org/10.1007/s10803-021-04890-4

Danforth, S. (2001). A pragmatic evaluation of three models of disability in special education. *Journal of Developmental and Physical Disabilities, 13*(4), 343–359. https://doi.org/10.1023/A:1012281312012

Darewych, O. H., Braganza, M. E., Newton, N. J., Kozman, K. H., & Argyle, H. (2020). Examining character strengths of developmental services workers in Canada: A mixed-methods pilot study. *Journal of Social Service Research*. Advance online publication. https://doi.org/10.1080/01488376.2020.1825586.

Datu, J., & Niemiec, R. M. (2023). *Disability: Character strengths, stigma, and acceptance across different disabilities*. Data from 21,800 people, collected on the VIA Institute on Character website.

Diener, E., Emmons, R. A., Larsen, R. J., & Griffin, S. (1985). The satisfaction with life scale. *Journal of Personality Assessment, 49*, 71–75. https://doi.org/10.1207/s15327752jpa4901_13

Dweck, C. (2006). *Mindset: The new psychology of success*. Random House.

Dykens, E. M. (2006). Toward a positive psychology of mental retardation. *American Journal of Orthopsychiatry, 76*(2), 185–193.

Emerson, E., Fortune, N., Llewellyn, G., & Stancliffe, R. (2021). Loneliness, social support, social isolation and wellbeing among working age adults with and without disability: Cross-sectional study. *Disability and Health Journal, 14*(1), 100965. https://doi.org/10.1016/j.dhjo.2020.100965

Gander, F., Proyer, R. T., Ruch, W., & Wyss, T. (2013). Strength-based positive interventions: Further evidence for their potential in enhancing well-being and alleviating depression. *Journal of Happiness Studies, 14*, 1241–1259. https://doi.org/10.1007/s10902-012-9380-0

Gilmore, L., & Cuskelly, M. (2014). Vulnerability to loneliness in people with intellectual disability: An explanatory model. *Journal of Policy and Practice in Intellectual Disabilities, 11*(3), 192–199. https://doi.org/10.1111/jppi.12089

Institute of Education Sciences. (2022). *Students with disabilities*. Accessed on October 3, 2022. Found at https://ies.ed.gov/.

Jach, H. K., Sun, J., Loton, D., Chin, T. C., & Waters, L. E. (2018). Strengths and subjective well-being in adolescence: Strength-based parenting and the moderating effect of mindset. *Journal of Happiness Studies, 19*, 567–586. https://doi.org/10.1007/s10902-016-9841-y

Kashdan, T. B., Blalock, D. V., Young, K. C., Machell, K. A., Monfort, S. S., McKnight, P. E., et al. (2018). Personality strengths in romantic relationships: Measuring perceptions of benefits and costs and their impact on personal and relational well-being. *Psychological Assessment, 30*, 241–258. https://doi.org/10.1037/pas0000464

Kirchner, J., Ruch, W., & Dziobek, I. (2016). Brief report: Character strengths in adults with autism spectrum disorder without intellectual impairment. *Journal of Autism and Developmental Disorders, 46*, 3330–3337. https://doi.org/10.1007/s10803-016-2865-7

Korn, M. A., Woodard, C. R., & Tucker, C. A. (2016). Positive character traits of special education staff: Commonalities and applications. *International Journal of Special Education, 31*(3).

Langer, E. (2006). *On becoming an artist: Reinventing yourself through mindful creativity*. Ballantine Books.

Linkins, M., Niemiec, R. M., Gillham, J., & Mayerson, D. (2014). Through the lens of strength: A framework for educating the heart. *Journal of Positive Psychology*. https://doi.org/10.1080/17439760.2014.888581

Linley, P. A., Nielsen, K. M., Gillett, R., & Biswas-Diener, R. (2010). Using signature strengths in pursuit of goals: Effects on goal progress, need satisfaction, and Well-being, and implications for coaching psychologists. *International Coaching Psychology Review, 5*(1), 6–15.

McGrath, R. E. (2015). Character strengths in 75 nations: An update. *Journal of Positive Psychology, 10*, 41–52. https://doi.org/10.1080/17439760.2014.888580

Meevissen, Y. M. C., Peters, M. L., & Alberts, H. J. E. M. (2011). Become more optimistic by imagining a best possible self: Effects of a two week intervention. *Journal of Behavior Therapy and Experimental Psychiatry, 42*, 371–378.

Mirenda, P., Zaidman-Zait, A., Cost, K. T., Smith, I. M., Zwaigenbaum, L., Duku, E., Kerns, C., Georgiades, S., Vaillancourt, T., Elsabbagh, M., Bennett, T., & Szatmari, P. (2022). Educators describe the "best things" about students with autism at school. *Journal of Autism and Developmental Disorders*. https://doi.org/10.1007/s10803-022-05761-2

Monterde, N., Blanco, I., & Hervas, G. (2022). Adaptation and incremental validity of the Pemberton happiness index: A new measure of integrative Well-being for people with intellectual disabilities. *Journal of Mental Health Research in Intellectual Disabilities*. https://doi.org/10.1080/19315864.2022.2098431

Naples, L. H., & Tuckwiller, E. D. (2021). Taking students on a strengths safari: A multidimensional pilot study of school-based wellbeing for young neurodiverse children. *International Journal of Environmental Research and Public Health, 18*. https://doi.org/10.3390/ijerph18136947

Niemiec, R. M. (2014). *Mindfulness and character strengths: A practical guide to flourishing*. Hogrefe.

Niemiec, R. M. (2018). *Character strengths interventions: A field-guide for practitioners*. Hogrefe.

Niemiec, R. M. (2019). Finding the golden mean: The overuse, underuse, and optimal use of character strengths. *Counseling Psychology Quarterly, 32*, 453–471. https://doi.org/10.1080/09515070.2019.1617674

Niemiec, R. M. (2020). Six functions of character strengths for thriving at times of adversity and opportunity: A theoretical perspective. *Applied Research in Quality of Life*. https://doi.org/10.1007/s11482-018-9692-2

Niemiec, R. M., & Pearce, R. (2021). The practice of character strengths: Unifying definitions, principles, and exploration of what's soaring, emerging, and ripe with potential in science and in practice. *Frontiers in Psychology, 11*, 590220. https://doi.org/10.3389/fpsyg.2020.590220

Niemiec, R. M., Shogren, K. A., & Wehmeyer, M. L. (2017). Character strengths and intellectual and developmental disability: A strengths-based approach from positive psychology. *Education and Training in Autism and Developmental Disabilities, 52*(1), 13.

Niemiec, R. M., Weinbrandt, D., Taylor, E., & Aunos, M. (2022). Mindfulness-based strengths practice—Access (MBSP-Access). A program and research process in development for people with intellectual/developmental disability.

Nocon, A. S., Roestorf, A., & Menéndeza, L. M. G. (2022). Positive psychology in neurodiversity: An investigation of character strengths in autistic adults in the United Kingdom in a community setting. *Research in Autism Spectrum Disorders, 99*. https://doi.org/10.1016/j.rasd.2022.102071

Otake, K., Shimai, S., Tanaka-Matsumi, J., Otsui, K., & Fredrickson, B. (2006). Happy people become happier through kindness: A counting kindness intervention. *Journal of Happiness Studies, 7*, 361–375.

Prasath, P. R., Morris, C., & Maccombs, S. (2021). Mindfulness-based strengths practice (MBSP) group intervention: A systematic review. *Journal of Counselor Practice, 12*(1), 1–22. https://doi.org/10.22229/asy1212021

Proyer, R. T., Ruch, W., & Buschor, C. (2013). Testing strengths-based interventions: A preliminary study on the effectiveness of a program targeting curiosity, gratitude, hope, humor, and zest for enhancing life satisfaction. *Journal of Happiness Studies, 14*(1), 275–292. https://doi.org/10.1007/s10902-012-9331-9

Quinlan, D., Vella-Brodrick, D. A., Gray, A., & Swain, N. (2019). Teachers matter: Student outcomes following a strengths intervention are mediated by teacher strengths spotting. *Journal of Happiness Studies, 20*, 2507–2523. https://doi.org/10.1007/s10902-018-0051-7

Raley, S. K., Shogren, K. A., & Cole, B. P. (2020). Positive psychology and education of students with disabilities: The way forward for assessment and intervention. *Advances in Neurodevelopmental Disorders*. https://doi.org/10.1007/s41252-020-00181-8

Ruch, W., Bakker, A. B., Tay, L., & Gander, F. (2022). *Handbook of positive psychology assessment*. Hogrefe.

Samson, A. C., & Antonelli, Y. (2013). Humor as character strength and its relation to life satisfaction and happiness in autism spectrum disorders. *Humor: International Journal of Humor Research, 26*(3), 477–491.

Schutte, N. S., & Malouff, J. M. (2019). The impact of signature character strengths interventions: A meta-analysis. *Journal of Happiness Studies, 20*, 1179–1196. https://doi.org/10.1007/s10902-018-9990-2

Schwartz, A. E. (2022, September 22). Personal communication.

Schwartz, A. E., Caoili, A., Beasley, J. B., Kramer, J. M., & Kalb, L. G. (2022). Clinical applications of the VIA inventory of strengths with individuals with intellectual/developmental disabilities. *Journal of Positive Psychology, 18*, 439.

Seligman, M. E. P., Steen, T. A., Park, N., & Peterson, C. (2005). Positive psychology progress: Empirical validation of interventions. *American Psychologist, 60*, 410–421. https://doi.org/10.1037/0003-066X.60.5.410

Shogren, K. A., Lopez, S. J., Wehmeyer, M. L., Little, T. D., & Pressgrove, C. L. (2006). The role of positive psychology constructs in predicting life satisfaction in adolescents with and without cognitive disabilities: An exploratory study. *Journal of Positive Psychology, 1*(1), 37–52.

Shogren, K. A., Wehmeyer, M. L., Forber-Pratt, A. J., & Palmer, S. B. (2015). *VIA inventory of strengths for youth (VIA-youth): Supplement for use when supporting youth with intellectual and developmental disabilities to complete the VIA-youth*. Kansas University Center on Developmental Disabilities.

Shogren, K. A., Gotto, G. S., Wehmeyer, M. L., Shaw, L., Seo, H., Palmer, S.,… Barton, K. N. (2016). The impact of the Self-Determined Career Development Model on self-determination outcomes. *Journal of Vocational Rehabilitation, 45*, 337–350. https://doi.org/10.3233/JVR-16083

Shogren, K. A., Singh, N., Niemiec, R. M., & Wehmeyer, M. (2017a). Character strengths and mindfulness. In M. Wehmeyer (Ed.), *Oxford handbooks online*. DOI: https://doi.org/10.1093/oxfordhb/9780199935291.013.77.

Shogren, K. A., Wehmeyer, M. L., Lang, K., Niemiec, R. M., & Seo, H. (2017b). The application of the VIA classification of strengths to youth with and without disabilities. *Inclusion, 5*(3), 213–228. https://doi.org/10.1352/2326-6988-5.3.213

Shogren, K. A., Shaw, L. A., Raley, S. K., Wehmeyer, M. L., Niemiec, R., & Adkins, M. (2018). Assessing character strengths in youth with intellectual disability: Reliability and factorial validity of the VIA-youth. *Intellectual and Developmental Disabilities, 56*(1), 13–29. https://doi.org/10.1352/1934-9556-56.1.13

Singh, N., Wahler, R., Adkins, A., & Myers, R. (2003). Soles of the feet: A mindfulness-based self-control intervention for aggression by an individual with mild mental retardation and mental illness. *Research in Developmental Disabilities, 24*. Retrieved from https://hsrc.himmelfarb.gwu.edu/smhs_psych_facpubs/748

Szucs, A., Schau, C., Muscara, K., & Tomasulo, D. (2019). Character strength activation for people with intellectual and developmental disabilities using video feedback in groups. *Journal of Education and Learning, 8*(1). https://doi.org/10.5539/jel.v8n1p12

Taylor, E. C., Livingston, L. A., Clutterbuck, R. A., Callan, M. J., & Shah, P. (2023). Psychological strengths and well-being: Strengths use predicts quality of life, well-being and mental health in autism. *Autism*. https://doi.org/10.1177/13623613221146440

Tomasulo, D. (2014). Positive group psychotherapy modified for adults with intellectual disabilities. *Journal of Intellectual Disabilities, 18*(4), 337–350. https://doi.org/10.1177/1744629514552153

Tomasulo, D., & Szucs, A. (2015). The ACTing cure: Evidence-based group treatment for people with intellectual disabilities. *Dramatherapy, 37*(2–3), 100–115. https://doi.org/10.1080/02630672.2016.1162824

Umucu, E., Lee, B., Genova, H. M., Chopik, W. J., Sung, C., Yasuoka, M., & Niemiec, R. M. (2022). Character strengths across disabilities: An international exploratory study and implications for positive psychiatry and psychology. *Frontiers in Psychiatry, 13*, 863977. https://doi.org/10.3389/fpsyt.2022.863977

VIA Institute on Character. (2022). *VIA assessments*. Found at: https://www.viacharacter.org/researchers/assessments. Accessed on 1 Sep 2022.

Vuorinen, K., Erikivi, A., & Uusitalo-Malmivaara, L. (2018). A character strength intervention in 11 inclusive Finnish classrooms to promote social participation of students with special education needs. *Journal of Research in Special Educational Needs*. https://doi.org/10.1111/1471-3802.12423

Wagner, L. (2018). Good character is what we look for in a friend: Character strengths are positively related to peer acceptance and friendship quality in early adolescents. *Journal of Early Adolescence*. https://doi.org/10.1177/0272431618791286

Wagner, L., Gander, F., Proyer, R. T., & Ruch, W. (2019). Character strengths and PERMA: Investigating the relationships of character strengths with a multidimensional framework of well-being. *Applied Research in Quality of Life, 15*, 307–328. https://doi.org/10.1007/s11482-018-9695-z

Walton, G. M., & Brady, S. T. (2017). The many questions of belonging. In A. J. Elliot, C. S. Dweck, & D. S. Yeager (Eds.), *Handbook of competence and motivation: Theory and application* (pp. 272–293). The Guilford Press.

Wehmeyer, M. L. (Ed.). (2013). *The Oxford handbook of positive psychology and disability*. Oxford University Press.

Wellenzohn, S., Proyer, R. T., & Ruch, W. (2016). Humor-based online positive psychology interventions: A randomized placebo-controlled long-term trial. *The Journal of Positive Psychology, 11*(6), 584–594. https://doi.org/10.1080/17439760.2015.1137624

Wilkinson, E., Vo, L. T. V., London, Z., Wilson, S., & Bal, V. H. (2022). Parent-reported strengths and positive qualities of adolescents and adults with autism spectrum disorder and/or intellectual disability. *Journal of Autism and Developmental Disorders*. https://doi.org/10.1007/s10803-021-05405-x

Woodard, C. (2009). Psychometric properties of the ASPeCT-DD: Measuring positive traits in persons with developmental disabilities. *Journal of Applied Research in Intellectual Disabilities, 27*, 433–444.

Yalom, I. (1995). *The theory and practice of group psychotherapy* (4th ed.). Basic Books.

Chapter 4
Character Strengths and Attention-Deficit/Hyperactivity Disorder (ADHD)

The Concepts

According to the Centers for Disease Control and Prevention (2022), the number of children ages 3–17 ever diagnosed with ADHD is 9.8%. Studies have shown that the prevalence of ADHD is at least as high among children in many countries outside the United States as in the U.S., and prevalence rates are highest when DSM diagnostic categories are used (Faraone et al., 2003). The prevalence of ADHD among US adults is 4.4%, considering data from 2003 (National Institute of Mental Health, 2003).

It is typical to start any discussion of ADHD emphasizing its two "D's"—deficit and disorder—and the symptoms and negative impact therein. We address the D's but start with what is needed in many ADHD contexts and the minds of many individuals—a character strengths-based, balanced perspective. From our review of numerous books and workbooks on ADHD from reputable authors and sources, the lack of exploration of activities, discussion, or insight into the internal capacities, character strengths, or other strengths is glaring. There are rare exceptions such as Giwerc (2011), who offers insights into the character strengths of adults with ADHD.

It is instructive to view the manifestations of ADHD as occurring on a continuum or a spectrum of more or less, as opposed to binary, all-or-none, abnormal versus normal functioning. This means that some aspects of ADHD may be unique strengths that are adaptive and positive (Archer, 2016; Sedgwick et al., 2019). Researchers have argued that increasing the understanding of positive expressions and outcomes of ADHD is important for decreasing stigmatization and in aiding psychoeducation and quality of life (Stolte et al., 2022). In addition, an enhanced awareness about the strengths of ADHD is suggested to help diagnosed individuals to embrace, accept, and manage their diagnosis and make better aligned choices for their educational and occupational life (Schippers et al., 2022). Indeed, ADHD researchers are emphasizing the importance of moving beyond diagnostic criteria

R. M. Niemiec, D. Tomasulo, *Character Strengths and Abilities Within Disabilities*, Positive Psychology and Disability Series,
https://doi.org/10.1007/978-3-031-36294-1_4

and studying ADHD in a broad, more balanced way that examines ability not only disability, and environmental facilitators not only environmental barriers (Mahdi et al., 2017). This balanced perspective mirrors movements in psychotherapy to look at strengths and deficits together (Rashid & Seligman, 2018).

When using the lens of a continuum model highlighting behavior as differences in degrees, it is important to acknowledge changes that occur by the context. The hyperactivity/zest expressed by a 10-year-old at home might be impairing as it irritates the siblings who are trying to do their homework; a couple of hours later when playing outside, the hyperactivity/zest becomes fun and engaging for playmates and manifests into leadership to organize an energizing sport activity.

Despite the applicability of the continuum model, the most common way to think about ADHD is through the lens of the medical model—generally accepted by the medical and psychological communities—framing ADHD according to the diagnostic criteria in the *DSM-5*. The criteria explain that children must meet six symptoms of inattention and/or hyperactivity/impulsivity (ages 17 and up must meet 5 symptoms). Examples of inattention symptoms include having trouble organizing tasks, easily distracted, forgetful in daily activities, careless mistakes, and avoidance/dislike of tasks requiring sustained mental effort. Examples of hyperactivity/impulsivity include being fidgety, acting as if "driven by a motor," talking excessively, blurting out answers before a question completes, and often interrupting/intruding on others.

In the *DSM-5*, ADHD is classified as a neurodevelopmental disorder and scientist Russell Barkley (2014) has extensively documented and reported the myriad of deficits associated with the disorder, namely, in executive functioning, such as the cognitive processes controlling movement, planning, organization, and inhibition control. He adds that because of the neurocognitive basis of this disorder, most individuals will be affected throughout the life span. Although ADHD is a problem in executive functioning, the science of executive functioning has failed to offer a consensual operational definition; the most common feature of scholars who have written on the concept is that executive functioning is self-regulation (Barkley, 2012). Thomas Brown (2013), a luminary ADHD scholar at Yale, offers a post-*DSM-5*, working definition of ADHD, noting it is "a complex syndrome of developmental impairments of executive functions, the self-management system of the brain, a system of mostly unconscious operations. These impairments are situationally variable, chronic, and significantly interfere with functioning in many aspects of the person's daily life" (p. 20). Brown outlines several executive functions impaired in ADHD including organizing and prioritizing (activation), focusing, sustaining, and shifting task attention (focus), regulating alertness, sustaining effort, and processing speed (effort), managing frustration and emotions (emotion), using working memory and accessing recall (memory), and monitoring and self-regulating (action). While these are deep neuropsychological elements, it is not difficult to wonder about the potential role of certain character strengths such as perseverance, prudence, social intelligence, and self-regulation.

In many ways, *difference* might be a better descriptor for ADHD than *disorder* as genetics and brain chemistry combine to impact differences in the transport/processing of the neurochemical dopamine and different reactions for each person to the environment (Archer, 2016).

The Science

In addition to some of the scholars' observations of strengths mentioned earlier (e.g., Archer, 2016), a handful of studies have looked at the strengths of adults with ADHD. Notably is Sedgwick et al. (2019) who offered a qualitative study of successful adults with ADHD and examined themes in comparison with the VIA classification. They aimed to examine the personal knowledge and lived experience of six adults by asking them about the advantages and disadvantages of having ADHD, a time when the ADHD helped them achieve something, and what they would miss if ADHD went away. The dominant findings of the study were six overarching themes of cognitive dynamism, courage, energy, humanity, resilience, and transcendence. On the surface, these align precisely with the virtues of the VIA Classification with only the virtues of justice and temperance not being present. The cognitive dynamism (and the sub-themes later described) connects closely with wisdom, courage and also energy (zest) and resilience (perseverance) align with the virtue of courage, and then humanity and transcendence are already listed as virtues.

To delve further into each overarching theme, Sedgwick et al. (2019) highlighted the cognitive dynamism sub-themes as divergent thinking, hyperfocus, creativity, and curiosity. Divergent thinking is aligned with the character strength of creativity while the participants' description of hyperfocus, akin to a flow state, is similar to the immersion and absorption in the character strength of love of learning. The sub-themes of courage were labeled as nonconformist, adventurousness, bravery, integrity, and persistence. Some of these were described as frequently feeling "different," feeling like an outsider, and overcoming struggles, being responsible for one's choices and risk-taking. The character strengths of bravery, perseverance, and honesty are directly reflected here. The other courage strength in the VIA classification is zest, which Sedgwick and colleagues describe as the larger theme of energy. The abundance of energy or zestful vitality is described with sub-themes of spirit, psychological, and physical. The sense of purpose and psychological will described by participants is reflective of the character strength of spirituality and bravery, respectively. The humanity theme contained thematic elements of self-acceptance, recognition of feelings, humor, and social intelligence. The latter two are actual character strengths and the recognition of feelings is viewed as a dimension of social intelligence in the VIA Classification (Peterson & Seligman, 2004). Self-acceptance was described by participants as tolerating oneself despite ADHD symptoms and functional impairments; this could be viewed as a quality of forgiveness—a letting go and forgiving oneself for one's limitations (Niemiec & McGrath, 2019). The resilience core theme contained subthemes of resilience and self-regulation, which are framed in the context of daily management of ADHD—emotionally, cognitively, and behaviorally. This core theme parallels Archer (2016) who describes resilience as an ADHD strength that manifests as an ability to be calm in a crisis, a propensity for multitasking, and a capacity for nonlinear thinking. The sixth core theme of Sedgwick and colleagues is transcendence and was noted as having the subtheme appreciation of beauty and excellence. It is likely the character strengths of gratitude and hope align with this theme as well. Arguably the strength categories least noted—directly or indirectly—are the justice virtue (teamwork, leadership, fairness) and temperance virtue (prudence, humility). This research shows substantial potential for the importance and alignment of character strengths and a positive perspective of ADHD to offer a more balanced perspective.

In a different study, Schippers et al. (2022) examined over 200 Dutch adults diagnosed with ADHD. They found a number of core themes including creativity, dynamism, flexibility, socio-affective skills, and higher-order cognitive skills. They found that some participants considered their impulsivity and hyperactivity to be a positive aspect in their life. These researchers reviewed their thematic findings with a focus group—a separate, additional group of individuals with ADHD—and these findings were confirmed along with additional consequences of living with ADHD, including being honest and open-minded. Again, the VIA character strengths are closely aligned with these important findings.

In a study that compared adults with ADHD and adults without ADHD on the VIA Survey, the adults without ADHD scored significantly higher on perseverance, prudence, and self-regulation (Ramsay et al., 2022). This research is consistent with the previous studies discussed as these three lower character strengths tended to be less highlighted and may be of particular concern for many people with ADHD. That is, in the other studies, there is a stronger emphasis on the specific character strengths (accounting for synonyms of character strengths) of creativity, judgment, honesty, perspective, zest. Other research has shown that ADHD is not connected with self-compassionate responding such as self-kindness, common humanity, and mindfulness, rather is significantly connected with non-self-compassionate responding, namely, self-criticism, isolation, and overidentification (Farmer et al., 2023). The latter uncompassionate self-responding fully mediated the relationship with well-being. These studies show that character strengths-and what might be the underuse of particular strengths-are important for understanding ADHD and some of the suffering experienced.

Research has also noted the importance of bringing a strengths-based approach to children with ADHD and interventions in school environments has been outlined by different research groups (Climie & Mastoras, 2015; McDougal et al., 2022). The positive characteristics of children/youth with ADHD has also been examined. Mahdi et al. (2017) examined 76 participants (individuals with ADHD, family members, professional caregivers), across five countries (i.e., Brazil, India, Saudi Arabia, South Africa, and Sweden), in a qualitative, semi-structured interview study. The most reported strengths were energy/drive, creativity, hyperfocus, agreeableness, empathy, and a willingness to help others. Using VIA character strengths language, these qualities would seem aligned with zest, creativity, kindness, and social intelligence.

Other studies have examined specific character strengths in isolation. The best example of this is the connection between creativity and ADHD. Creative thinking, creative style, and creative achievements have been studied in people with ADHD. One study found that ADHD symptoms in the general adult population were associated with higher divergent thinking and predicted divergent thinking up to a certain level of symptomatology (Stolte et al., 2022). Other studies have found that adults with ADHD outperform adults without ADHD on creativity measures; this has been shown on standardized measures and real-world creative achievements (White & Shah, 2011).

In examining the preceding early findings alongside the VIA Classification of 24 character strengths, it would seem the category least accounted for is the temperance category (which contains the character strengths of self-regulation, prudence, forgiveness, and humility). As this category is viewed as the self-control strengths and ADHD is often characterized as involving a lack of inhibition or a lack of self-control, it is logical that these particular character strengths may be important themes for understanding ADHD.

Learning Disability

The number of children with ADHD who also have a learning disability is estimated to be between 20% and 30% (Learning Disabilities Association of America, 2023). Because of this high comorbidity between ADHD and learning disabilities - and their falling in the same DSM-5 category of neurodevelopmental disorders-we offer this additional section devoted to learning disabilities. We briefly note a couple studies that have looked at both conditions, and in the practice section that follows, we offer a case example of character strengths applied to a person with both conditions.

A learning disability refers to a problem involved with learning through spoken or written language, arithmetic/calculation, or reasoning/integration of ideas, and most typically revolves around reading, writing, spelling, or math. Individuals with learning disabilities and ADHD may have similar knowledge in learning skills, however, the approach to learning tasks are distinct and thereby different approaches are needed for each (Reaser et al., 2007). That said, it has been suggested that tapping into self-efficacy and authenticity is important for both ADHD and learning disability (Costello & Stone, 2012).

One study looked at a small sample of students with learning disabilities and/or ADHD. It found that students experienced positive benefits in completing a program that involved identifying and using strengths among other practices in self-determination and positivepsychology (Farmer et al., 2015).

The Practice

All of the examples and practices discussed in this section could be adapted for children or adults with ADHD. We are targeting the use and practice of *character strengths* for people with ADHD, but as discussed in Chap. 1, there are many other categories of strength that can (and should) also be targeted such as the person's skills, interests, talents, and resources.

As many practitioners report, it is crucial to help counteract the individual's entrenched negativity bias to help people identify what is good, and learn to channel or harness character strengths to flourish, overcome adversity, and to lead a full and meaningful life. It is in this spirit by which we offer this section.

The precise integrating of character strengths with ADHD is in need of evidence-based interventions for child and adult populations. To inform future research and contribute foundational practices for practitioners, we offer strategies based in theoretical work (e.g., Niemiec, 2018), the science discussed in the previous section, the larger science of character strengths (e.g., VIA Institute, 2023), and the practice of character strengths and character strengths interventions (Niemiec & Pearce, 2021).

We suggest the exploration—scientifically and practically—of four general areas of application:

1. Integrating character strengths into existing ADHD treatments/approaches
2. Targeting character strengths of clients
3. Deploying character strengths interventions
4. Using character strengths (the practitioner using their own strengths)

We discuss practical concepts and application for each of these areas.

Integrating Character Strengths into Existing ADHD Treatments/Approaches

In terms of the treatment, support, and care of people with ADHD, the deployment or integration of character strengths has not been a focus. Rather, the traditional, evidence-based approach is pharmacological. The gold standard approach for serious cases of ADHD (among typically developing children/teens) is a combination of medication and behavior therapy. For the latter, a number of practical parent training programs have shown to be helpful for behavioral problems including parent–child interaction therapy (PCIT), parent management training (PMT), positive parenting program (Triple P), and research units in behavioral intervention (RUBI). There are a number of behavioral strategies (for adults with ADHD and for parents of children with ADHD) which include keeping a routine, managing distractions, self-monitoring, chunking tasks and activities, praising good behaviors, using clear and specific language, developing positive experiences, using choices, and attending to healthy living such as creating good habits with eating, exercise, and sleep.

These approaches—pharmacological, behavioral, and parent training—can benefit from weaving in character strengths. Character strengths are not mutually exclusive from these approaches. For example, a medical or psychological practitioner supporting clients in taking medicine for ADHD can deliberately encourage, call-out, and work with different character strengths to enhance adherence.

- The strength of self-regulation to self-monitor one's dosage and use each day. The client (or parent) tracks the usage on their smart-device or self-monitoring form.

- The strength of prudence to think through a particular plan for medicine use. Many successful plans will link with environmental cues, such as putting the medicine in a place where the individual passes by around the time they need to take it and linking it with a meal or other routinized action.
- The strength of hope to share the positive benefits and expectations of successful adherence. Hope was a significant predictor of medication adherence among asthma patients between 8 and 12 (Berg, et al., 2007).
- The strength of judgment/critical thinking to analyze the costs and benefits of taking the medicine. One obstacle to adherence is the individual's concern about side effects. This *cost* can be laid out next to the potential *benefits* of taking it, as well as the *cost* of not taking it and the *benefits* of not taking it. This four-quadrant approach encourages balanced and critical thinking about the treatment approach.

The direct callout of these or other character strengths successfully deployed in these instances and/or the labeling of that strength to be used that week/month can be an empowering frame for clients.

In parent training groups for parents of children with ADHD, the deploying of character strengths in different ways can have a positive effect. The following are seven examples practitioners might use in group experiences; the strategy of that use is noted in parentheses:

- That behavioral strategy of reinforcement that you used with your child this week was really well done. It seems like you used quite a bit of *creativity* to figure out ways to make it work with your schedule! (spotting the character strength used).
- I notice you show a lot of *curiosity* in this group by asking questions and exploring different topics. Have you reflected on ways you can use your curiosity when your child shows disruptive symptoms? (targeting the strength of the parent).
- I see that you are high in the strength of *perspective* which means to take stock in the bigger picture of life and parenting, as opposed to getting lost in the detail of one symptom in the moment. How might you remind yourself of this incredible character strength throughout your parenting days? (encouraging the parent's future use of the strength).
- Each time you share about your parenting of your child, I am struck by your strength of *love* which drives everything you do and your *gratitude* as you pause to appreciate your life and your connection with your child (general reinforcement of a pattern of strengths use).
- I understand you are wanting to set a goal to spend a structured amount of one-on-one time with you child for 20 min each day. Which of your *character strengths* will help you successfully accomplish this goal? (pointing out character strengths as pathways to any goal).
- Let us look at your highest strengths of character—your most core and best qualities as a human being. Surely, each of these *(signature) strengths* are critical in your parenting, right? They involve your being authentic and true in your relationship with your child. How might you be sure to bring these *signature strengths* forward each day as a parent? (highlighting the importance of the parent's signature strengths).

- You have dealt with a lot of unique stressors this week. That has taken a toll on your parenting and the behavioral strategies you wanted to prioritize this week. I also want to point out that you displayed substantial *perseverance* to overcoming the obstacles and problems and still getting everything done, and being here today to discuss it! (validating the parent's suffering and struggles while infusing strengths use).

Note that none of these strategies require the practitioner to change their treatment protocol or adopt a new approach. As discussed in Niemiec (2018), character strengths can be woven into any theoretical orientation or psychological approach and the foundation and theory of that approach or program need not be restructured.

Adaptation of Existing Programs for ADHD

Another integration lens for ADHD is to consider programs that have not been studied for people specifically with ADHD but are evidenced-based. Such programs—if rationale and application can be devised for ADHD—might be ripe with opportunity to be adapted and studied for ADHD. One character strengths program that has good evidence is Mindfulness-Based Strengths Practice (MBSP; Niemiec, 2023). MBSP is an 8-week, manualized program, applied to the general public and to practitioners (usually adults), involving the integration of the latest science and best practices of character strengths and of mindfulness. While some research has shown mindfulness programs for ADHD shows good potential to be beneficial (Mitchell et al., 2015; van de Weijer-Bergsma et al., 2012), the integration with character strengths has not been studied formally. The value-add of character strengths to mindfulness interventions, however, has been shown to be substantial, as evidenced by three studies in which MBSP was superior to the most popular mindfulness program (Hofmann et al., 2019; Monzani et al., 2021; Pang & Ruch, 2019).

As MBSP emphasizes improvement in the self-regulation of attention and development of curiosity, openness, and acceptance, there is emphasis on bringing mindfulness into daily actions like eating, listening, walking, and working that are normally taken for granted. The emphasis on mindful strengths awareness, exploration, and application in domains of life, goal-setting, relationship-building, stress management, and managing strengths overuse/underuse in different contexts are overarching points of emphasis that can be readily applied to ADHD.

A formal adaptation of MBSP for ADHD might include an infusion of approaches involving movement, bite-size lecture/input portions, and expansion of discussion about personal character strengths use. While MBSP has been most often applied to adults, emerging evidence points to benefits for teens and young college students (Park, 2020).

Overall, the integration of character strengths in standard ADHD treatment approaches would seem to be a straightforward way for enhancing adherence, facilitating relationship building, and aligned with offering empowering tools to the client and family.

Integration with Health Habits

As mentioned earlier, optimizing physical health in terms of lifestyle adjustment and healthy living is an important component of ADHD management. Niemiec (2019b) has offered 5 core pillars of health—healthy eating/drinking, sleeping, exercise/movement, socializing, and self-care—and emphasized the importance of character strengths as foundational pathways for each. In a study with 60,000 individuals, researchers found the character strengths of zest, hope, self-regulation, and gratitude were of primary importance for physical health areas (Weziak-Bialowolska et al., 2023). An intentional focus on these character strengths might provide a streamlined dual-benefit—physically and psychologically—for people with ADHD.

Targeting Character Strengths of Clients

Considering the research in the science section of this chapter, practitioners can be on the lookout for identifying and discussing character strengths that might be strong for many people with ADHD. The character strengths of creativity, zest, humor, curiosity, perspective, and bravery are good starting points for these discussions. Practitioners can deploy the classic, character strengths model—the aware, explore, apply model (Niemiec, 2018, 2023)—to target any character strength and give a framework for the discussion. For example, practitioners can use the following questions, if applied to the strength of zest:

- *Aware*: Where is zest in your character strengths profile (your rank-order of strengths from 1 to 24)? Do you identify with this character strength as a part of you? Please explain.
- *Explore*: When have you used your strength of zest to help you at a time of stress? Which situations are you most likely to turn to your zest? What does zest look like when you are using it strongly and adaptively? How do you increase your zest when you actually need it? How might zest help you with an ADHD symptom?
- *Apply*: What might be a strategy for using your zest in a way that helps you and others? Might we discuss an action plan for daily use of zest?
- Practitioners can also apply a deliberate, evidence-based intervention for any particular strength. Here are a few examples taken from Niemiec (2018):
- *Creativity*: Develop divergent thinking, which means to generate multiple alternate solutions, instead of searching for one "correct" solution (Scott et al., 2004). After you name a problem, brainstorm a list of ideas of potential solutions.
- *Curiosity*: Consider an activity that you dislike. Pay attention to three novel features of this activity while you do it (Langer, 2006).
- *Perspective*: Have a conversation with a wise person (or imagine the conversation). If imagined, visualize the full dialogue in terms of questions asked, responses given, the nuances of the discussion, and any advice that would be offered (Baltes & Staudinger, 2000). This boosts wisdom-related knowledge.

- *Bravery*: Focus on the outcomes of courageous acts; for example, thinking of the person being helped, reminding oneself of the goodness of the action, or thinking about an obligation to act (Pury, 2008).
- *Zest*: Going outside, especially in nature, boosts zest and vitality (Ryan et al., 2010). Individuals can be encouraged to take breaks outdoors and arrange their day to spend some time in nature.
- *Humor*: At the end of each day for the next week, write down the three funniest things you experienced or did and explain why those things happened (Gander et al., 2013).

Deploying Character Strengths Interventions

There are a large number of character strengths interventions (see manuals by Niemiec, 2018, 2023) that could be studied and adapted to align to help people with ADHD. A few examples of interventions that could be deployed include using a signature strength in a new way, character strengths appreciation, and character strengths alignment. In many ways, each of the subsections of this practice section are a form of a character strengths intervention.

Discussions of character strengths overuse, underuse, and optimal-use offer a lens of understanding and management of strengths (Niemiec, 2019a); these can be further enhanced with the tempering effect (managing an overused strength) and the towing effect (boosting up a lower strength) as theorized in Niemiec (2020). While the examination of clusters of overused and underused strengths has been examined in the context of deepening understanding of psychological disorders such as social anxiety disorder (Freidlin et al., 2017) and obsessive-compulsive disorder (Littman-Ovadia & Freidlin, 2019), overuse/underuse/optimal use models have not been studied in the context of ADHD at the time of this writing. Based on the discussions in this chapter, the reader might begin to draw potential hypotheses such as the overuse of zest, creativity, and curiosity and the underuse of prudence and self-regulation. Such combinations vary by context and individual and empirical research is needed to examine these areas.

Reframing or positive reappraisal is another intervention that is important to explore in the context of ADHD. To reframe is to change the conversation, to shift the mindset, to look more holistically at the individual, to empower oneself, and in many cases to look more realistically. A first-line question emerges—what strength is present in this behavior? It might be a strength that is causing the experience or manifesting in a way that is not precisely aligned with the environmental demands and expectations. It might represent an overuse or an underuse of strengths in the situation (Niemiec, 2019a). Knowing the potential character strengths at play—regardless of the level of contextual imbalance—can offer a "language" for client insight and reframing. We consider the 3 classic ADHD symptom clusters—inattention, hyperactivity, and impulsivity—and two examples of character strengths use expressed as a symptom therein; with these examples, we do not delve into interpretations of overuse and underuse which could also be perceived and used in the reframing context.

Table 4.1 Examples of character strength reframes for conventional ADHD symptoms

ADHD cluster	adhd symptom	Character strength	Reframe example
Inattention	Trouble holding attention on tasks	Curiosity	Jeff is curious of so many topics and activities that he often hops from one thing to another
	Doesn't listen when spoken to	Perseverance	Bayden is often absorbed and sticking with the task at hand—he focuses on video games and reading adventure books; he overcomes obstacles and anything in the way (such as people telling him to stop!)
Hyperactivity	Fidgety—tapping hands/feet	Creativity	Caden often has a new idea he would like to share, especially at team meetings; when he thinks of it, he starts to tap his feet and fidget with his pens, eager to share the new ideas and insights with others
	Acts as if driven by a motor	Zest	Monique acts as though she is in a perpetual state of excitement and happy energy—her zest comes through most in her sport activities and social interactions
Impulsivity	Trouble waiting for one's turn	Bravery	Jonah has a fear of disappointing or upsetting others but he readily taps his bravery by overcoming that fear and skipping line at recess which risks upsetting others
	Interrupts others	Love of learning	Sandy is eager to discuss and explore a range of topics, so she sometimes finishes people's sentences. She realizes this so she uses her strength of fairness and lets others finish her sentences as well!

Table 4.1 is not intended to offer a replacement for a diagnosis, symptom, or cluster. It is shown as an addition to ADHD language. These reframes help the practitioner to see the human being in the experience and to not get lost in deficit-based thinking.

Using Character Strengths (The Practitioner Using their Own Strengths)

A final important area to consider is the character strengths of the professional (or parent) offering support to someone with ADHD, adult or child.

In discussing character strengths with professionals, parents, and individuals with ADHD, we composed a table of examples consisting of one way each character strength can be deliberately used by the individual helping someone with ADHD (see Table 4.2).

Table 4.2 Ways a practitioner (or parent) can use any character strength to support someone with ADHD. Limited to one behavioral example per strength

Character strength	Example of practitioner's own strength use (Limited to 1 per strength)
Creativity	Point out that there are many possible ways of solving a problem
Curiosity	When in doubt, ask a question, especially when a pattern of problematic behavior is manifesting
Judgment/critical thinking	Politely offer different views when the person is stuck in one way of thinking about something
Love of learning	Appeal directly to the person's capacity to learn—to learn about themselves, about ways to thrive, and optimal health and treatment approaches
Perspective	Offer advice based on one's own experience and observations in a supportive way
Bravery	Despite the intensity of an individual's actions or words, turn to bravery to challenge, redirect, or discuss the situation
Perseverance	Persevere with spotting and appreciating character strengths due to the pervasiveness of deficit-based propensities of individuals
Honesty	Give your direct opinion on a treatment or strategy that does not appear to be working well
Zest	Join the individual by expressing similar enthusiasm in an appropriate situation
Love	Offer the warmth and genuineness of quality listening to the individual. Give your full presence to them in a given situation
Kindness	Encourage the person to practice self-kindness—being more kind to themselves after a mistake
Social intelligence	Express empathy when the person has a setback with their reactivity and impulsiveness
Teamwork	Take a team approach. Discuss how you and the individual might work together as a team to help them with something.
Fairness	In a situation in which you do not agree with the person, try fairness as an approach that allows for their opinion
Leadership	Organize an activity or shared task that the individual struggles with or tends to not organize. Role model your leadership with it
Forgiveness	Practice internally "letting go" when a minor reactive comment or behavior occurs
Humility	Role model an approach of being grounded and centered that can serve as a trusting anchor for the person
Prudence	Offer ideas for planning an evening or weekend and take action to carry out each step
Self-regulation	Practice mindful breathing together. Practice bringing the wandering mind back to the breath each time a distraction emerges. Consider a daily or weekly practice together
Appreciation of beauty	Go for a walk outside and point out the beauty seen in the sky, buildings, trees, or people
Gratitude	Express thankfulness to the person for the character strength they displayed today. Explain why you are grateful for that strength expressed
Hope	Verbally express hope for the person's future, emphasizing your optimism and positive expectations, which might be received as a pleasant surprise

(continued)

Table 4.2 (continued)

Character strength	Example of practitioner's own strength use (Limited to 1 per strength)
Humor	Laugh with the person. Watch shows together—on the television or in-person—in which laughter is expected
Spirituality	Appreciate the sacredness of any given moment with the person—in a conversation or other shared experience

Some strategies in Table 4.2 might be more suited for adults or for children. The table can serve as a catalyst for parents and professionals to remember there are far more things going right with themselves and the individual they are supporting than what is wrong with them. The character strengths provide a language for understanding that. While any of the strategies listed in the table can be useful to anyone, these are particularly applicable to supporting many of the common struggles akin to ADHD.

Case Example

Hannah was a university student who experienced both ADHD and a learning disability. She attended a weekly tutoring program to help her with her learning and planning in the classroom and in doing homework.

One day during the tutoring session, Hannah showed an additional degree of tension and struggle. The tutor observed this in Hannah and they had the following conversation.

Hannah (looks down): *I just can't do it!*

Tutor: *What is it, Hannah?*

Hannah (hits the table with her fist): *I don't know. This math assignment is just too hard. I don't get it!*

Tutor: *It's OK, we can figure it out together. Is everything else alright?*

Hannah (fidgeting): *Yes, I'm fine. I don't understand this stuff. I feel like I'm never going to figure out anything in this class.*

Tutor: *Can we stop for a moment where I can share something with you?*

Hannah (fidgeting): *Fine.*

Tutor: *I would like to point out that I perceive you to be one of the most brave people I have ever met. And perseverant too.*

Hannah (stops fidgeting, makes eye contact): *What?*

Tutor: *Day after day you go to class knowing that there will be challenges and confusion and upsetting emotions, but you keep going. You face those difficult feelings. You know that some kids and even some teachers won't be particularly accepting of you or helpful. And some will be downright mean. But you go anyway. You handle those adversities. That is bravery. That inspires me. And, you go forth trying your best in each class and each social interaction. You overcome every obstacle doing what you can. Now that is perseverance. You are one of the most brave and perseverant people I have met.*

This conversation involving honest strengths-spotting by the tutor helped to open Hannah's eyes to her inner capacities. These were capacities she had forgotten and had not been using deliberately. They were capacities that no person had ever directly pointed out in her before. With a perspective-building conversation like this, it was no problem for Hannah to realize she had more than enough inner resources to be able to handle the small task of trying a bit harder on an assignment. Moreover, it was a conversation she held in her heart for years—and many adversities—to come.

Future Directions

In some ways, much of the content in this chapter is a set of considerations for future research. The science of character strengths for ADHD is in its infancy and several studies have been shared to build upon. The practices discussed can be studied with ADHD populations from the perspective of both incremental benefit (does adding character strengths to an existing treatment approach or program provide additional benefit?) and standalone benefit (what benefit does a particular character strengths intervention or character strengths program tailored to ADHD bring to individuals?).

There are a number of areas discussed in this chapter that we view to hold exciting potential, including the adaptation of MBSP for adults (or young people) with ADHD; the examination of strength overuse and underuse patterns to identify, explain, and eventually provide intervention support for people with ADHD; and said simply, to see randomized character strengths intervention studies to boost well-being or manage stress in people with ADHD, to name a few areas.

Key Takeaways

- ADHD is a common condition with dominant treatment approaches emphasizing a deficit-based approach. A continuum model—viewing ADHD behaviors on a spectrum—has been espoused as a more balanced approach with strength-based possibilities. ADHD, in many ways, is better captured as a *difference* as opposed to a disorder.
- As a neurodevelopmental disorder, ADHD has been framed as a problem in executive functioning of which self-regulation is a central component.
- Some researchers have begun to look at specific character strengths in people with ADHD such as creativity, while others have conducted interviews with people with ADHD and highlighted nearly all 24 character strengths as important, such as strengths of cognitive dynamism, courage, energy, humanity, resilience, and transcendence.
- From a practical perspective, character strengths can be integrated into any existing ADHD treatment approach. It is hypothesized that this would provide a value-add to well-being and adversity management.
- There are substantial opportunities for interventions involving the targeting of character strengths in clients, the deploying of strong character strengths interventions, and the use of the practitioner's own character strengths as part of their approach.

References

Archer, D. (2016). The ADHD advantage: What you thought was a diagnosis may be your greatest strength. Avery.

Baltes, P. B., & Staudinger, U. (2000). Wisdom: A metaheuristic (pragmatic) to orchestrate mind and virtue toward excellence. *American Psychologist, 55*, 122–136. https://doi.org/10.1037/0003-066X.55.1.122

Barkley, R. A. (2012). *Executive functions: What they are, how they work, and why they evolved.* Guilford.

Barkley, R. A. (2014). *Attention-deficit hyperactivity disorder,* 4th edn. *A handbook for diagnosis and treatment.* Guilford.

Berg, C. J., Rapoff, M. A., Snyder, C. R., & Belmont, J. M. (2007). The relationship of children's hope to pediatric asthma treatment adherence. *Journal of Positive Psychology, 2*, 176–184.

Brown, T. E. (2013). *A new understanding of ADHD in children and adults: Executive function impairments.* Routledge.

Centers for Disease Control and Prevention. (2022). *Data and statistics about ADHD.* https://www.cdc.gov/ncbddd/adhd/data.html. Accessed on January 15, 2023.

Climie, E. A., & Mastoras, S. M. (2015). ADHD in schools: Adopting a strengths-based perspective. *Canadian Psychology, 56*(3), 295–300. https://doi.org/10.1037/cap0000030

Costello, C. A., & Stone, S. L. M. (2012). Positive psychology and self-efficacy: Potential benefits for college students with attention deficit hyperactivity disorder and learning disabilities. *Journal of Postsecondary Education and Disability, 25*(2), 119–129.

Faraone, S. V., Sergeant, J., Gillberg, C., & Biederman, J. (2003). The worldwide prevalence of ADHD: is it an American condition? *World Psychiatry, 2*(2), 104–113.

Farmer, J. L., Allsopp, D. H., & Ferron, J. M. (2015). Impact of the personal strengths program on self-determination levels of college students with LD and/or ADHD. *Learning Disability Quarterly, 38*(3), 145–159.

Farmer, G. M., Ohan, J. L., Finlay-Jones, A. L., & Bayliss, D. M. (2023). Well-being and distress in university students with ADHD traits: The mediating roles of self-compassion and emotion regulation difficulties. *Mindfulness, 14*, 448–459. https://doi.org/10.1007/s12671-022-02051-x

Freidlin, P., Littman-Ovadia, H., & Niemiec, R. M. (2017). Positive psychopathology: Social anxiety via character strengths underuse and overuse. *Personality and Individual Differences, 108*, 50–54. https://doi.org/10.1016/j.paid.2016.12.003

Gander, F., Proyer, R. T., Ruch, W., & Wyss, T. (2013). Strength-based positive interventions: Further evidence for their potential in enhancing well-being and alleviating depression. *Journal of Happiness Studies, 14*, 1241–1259. https://doi.org/10.1007/s10902-012-9380-0

Giwerc, D. (2011). *Permission to proceed: The keys to creating a life of passion, purpose and possibility for adults with ADHD.* Vervante.

Hofmann, J., Heintz, S., Pang, D., & Ruch, W. (2019). Differential relationships of light and darker forms of humor with mindfulness. *Applied Research in Quality of Life., 15*, 369. https://doi.org/10.1007/s11482-018-9698-9

Langer, E. (2006). *On becoming an artist: Reinventing yourself through mindful creativity.* Ballantine Books.

Learning Disabilities Association of America. (2023). *ADHD.* https://ldaamerica.org/disabilities/adhd/. Accessed on 15 Jan 2023.

Littman-Ovadia, H., & Freidlin, P. (2019). Positive psychopathology and positive functioning: OCD, flourishing and satisfaction with life through the lens of character strength underuse, overuse and optimal use. *Applied Research in Quality of Life, 15*, 529. https://doi.org/10.1007/s11482-018-9701-5

Mahdi, S., Vijoen, M., Massuti, R., Selb, M., Almodayfer, O., Karande, S., de Vries, P. J., Rohde, L., & Bölte, S. (2017). An international qualitative study of ability and disability in ADHD using the WHO-ICF framework. *European Child and Adolescent Psychiatry, 26*(10), 1219–1231.

McDougal, E., Tai, C., Stewart, T. M., Booth, J. N., & Rhodes, S. M. (2022). Understanding and supporting attention deficit hyperactivity disorder (ADHD) in the primary school classroom: Perspectives of children with ADHD and their teachers. *Journal of Autism and Developmental Disorders*. https://doi.org/10.1007/s10803-022-05639-3

Mitchell, J. T., Zylowska, L., & Kollins, S. H. (2015). Mindfulness meditation training for attention-deficit/hyperactivity disorder in adulthood: Current empirical support, treatment overview, and future directions. *Cognitive and Behavioral Practice, 22*(2), 172–191. https://doi.org/10.1016/j.cbpra.2014.10.002

Monzani, L., Escartin, J., Ceja, L., & Bakker, A. B. (2021). Blending mindfulness practices and character strengths increases employee wellbeing: A second-order meta-analysis and a follow-up field experiment. *Human Resource Management Journal., 31*, 1025. https://doi.org/10.1111/1748-8583.12360

National Institute of Mental Health. (2003). *Attention-deficit/hyperactivity disorder (ADHD).* https://www.nimh.nih.gov/health/statistics/attention-deficit-hyperactivity-disorder-adhd. Accessed on 15 Jan 2023.

Niemiec, R. M. (2018). *Character strengths interventions: A field-guide for practitioners*. Hogrefe.

Niemiec, R. M. (2019a). Finding the golden mean: The overuse, underuse, and optimal use of character strengths. *Counselling Psychology Quarterly, 32*(3–4), 453–471. https://doi.org/10.1080/09515070.2019.161767400

Niemiec, R. M. (2019b). *The strengths-based workbook for stress relief.* New Harbinger.

Niemiec, R. M. (2020). Six functions of character strengths for thriving at times of adversity and opportunity: A theoretical perspective. *Applied Research in Quality of Life, 15*, 551–572. https://doi.org/10.1007/s11482-018-9692-2

Niemiec, R. M. (2023). *Mindfulness and character strengths: A practitioner's guide to MBSP* (2nd ed.). Hogrefe.

Niemiec, R. M., & McGrath, R. E. (2019). *The power of character strengths: Appreciate and ignite your positive personality*. VIA Institute on Character.

Niemiec, R. M., & Pearce, R. (2021). The practice of character strengths: Unifying definitions, principles, and exploration of what's soaring, emerging, and ripe with potential in science and in practice. *Frontiers in Psychology, 11*, 590220. https://doi.org/10.3389/fpsyg.2020.590220

Pang, D., & Ruch, W. (2019). Fusing character strengths and mindfulness interventions: Benefits for job satisfaction and performance. *Journal of Occupational Health Psychology, 24*(1), 150–162. https://doi.org/10.1037/ocp0000144

Park, R. J. (2020). *Mindfulness-based strengths practice: A 'toolbox' for self-efficacy in higher education*. Dissertation for University of Lincoln.

Peterson, C., & Seligman, M. E. P. (2004). *Character strengths and virtues: A handbook and classification*. Oxford University Press and American Psychological Association.

Pury, C. L. S. (2008). Can courage be learned? In S. J. Lopez (Ed.), *Positive psychology: Exploring the best in people* (*Discovering human strengths*) (Vol. 1, pp. 109–130). Praeger.

Ramsay, J. R., Giwerc, D., McGrath, R. E., & Niemiec, R. M. (2022). Are there strengths associated with adult ADHD? Comparison of adults with ADHD and Controls on the VIA inventory of strengths. Manuscript submitted for publication.

Rashid, T., & Seligman, M. E. P. (2018). *Positive psychotherapy: Clinician manual*. Oxford University Press.

Reaser, A., Prevatt, F., Petscher, Y., & Proctor, B. (2007). The learning and study strategies of college students with ADHD. *Psychology in the Schools, 44*, 627–638. https://doi.org/10.1002/pits.20252

Ryan, R. M., Weinstein, N., Bernstein, J., Brown, K. W., Mistretta, L., & Gagné, M. (2010). Vitalizing effects of being outdoors and in nature. *Journal of Environmental Psychology, 30*, 159–168. https://doi.org/10.1016/j.jenvp.2009.10.009

Schippers, L. M., Horstman, L. I., Velde, H. V., Pereira, R. R., Zinkstok, J., Mostert, J. C., Greven, C. U., & Hoogman, M. (2022). A qualitative and quantitative study of self-reported positive characteristics of individuals with ADHD. *Frontiers in Psychiatry, 12*. https://doi.org/10.3389/fpsyt.2022.922788

Scott, G., Leritz, L. E., & Mumford, M. D. (2004). The effectiveness of creativity training: A quantitative review. *Creativity Research Journal, 16*(4), 361–388. https://doi.org/10.1080/10400410409534549

Sedgwick, J. A., Merwood, A., & Asherson, P. (2019). The positive aspects of attention deficit hyperactivity disorder: A qualitative investigation of successful adults with ADHD. *ADHD Attention Deficit Hyperactivity Disorders, 11*, 241–253. https://doi.org/10.1007/s12402-018-0277-6

Stolte, M., Trindade-Pons, V., Vlaming, P., Jakobi, B., Franke, B., Kroesbergen, E. H., Baas, M., & Hoogman, M. (2022). Characterizing creative thinking and creative achievements in relation to symptoms of attention-deficit/hyperactivity disorder and autism spectrum disorder. *Frontiers in Psychiatry, 13*. https://doi.org/10.3389/fpsyt.2022.909202

van de Weijer-Bergsma, E., Formsma, A. R., & de Bruin, E. I. (2012). The effectiveness of mindfulness training on behavioral problems and attentional functioning in adolescents with ADHD. *Journal of Child and Family Studies, 21*, 775–787. https://doi.org/10.1007/s10826-011-9531-7

VIA Institute. (2023). *What the research says about character strengths*. Available at: https://www.viacharacter.org/research/findings. Accessed 2 Jan 2023.

Weziak-Bialowolska, D., Bialowolski, P., & Niemiec, R. M. (2023). Character strengths and health-related quality of life in a large international sample: A cross-sectional analysis. *Journal of Research in Personality, 103*, 104338. https://doi.org/10.1016/j.jrp.2022.104338

White, H. A., & Shah, P. (2011). Creative style and achievement in adults with attention-deficit/hyperactivity disorder. *Personality and Individual Differences, 50*(5), 673–677. https://doi.org/10.1016/j.paid.2010.12.015

Chapter 5
Trauma Disabilities and Character Strengths

The Woman Going Blind. ~Rainer Maria Rilke
She sat much like the others taking tea.
At first, the way she held her cup seemed just a little different from all the rest.
One time she smiled. That almost hurt to see.
And when at last we stood up, chatting on, and, as the impulse took us, slowly walked through many other rooms (we laughed and talked), I watched her there.
She followed where they'd gone, like one who in a little while must rise to sing before a crowd, a bit withdrawn, the light from outside, as upon a pond, shining on her bright, rejoicing eyes.

She followed slowly, letting time pass by, as if some hindrance had to be transcended, and yet as if, when the transition ended, she would no longer go on foot, but fly.

The Concepts

In the past two decades the swell of literature on trauma has amplified our understanding of what qualifies as a traumatic event, why these events are responded to differently by different people, and how some potentially traumatic experiences can be an accelerant for growth and well-being. This chapter takes a more specific look at the many roles character strengths might play in predicting how well individuals manage, cope with, and/or transcend traumatic experiences.

The number of people who are disabled, meaning not able to function fully because of a physical, psychological, or behavioral barrier, fluctuates daily, yet a consistent percentage of the population is always struggling. To illustrate, approximately 26% (1 in 4) of people in the United States have a disability with 40% over the age of 65 reporting disabling conditions. The World Health Organization notes everyone will experience a disability in their lifetime making disability a human

R. M. Niemiec, D. Tomasulo, *Character Strengths and Abilities Within Disabilities*, Positive Psychology and Disability Series,
https://doi.org/10.1007/978-3-031-36294-1_5

rights issue—and reports there are a billion people (including over 93 million children and 720 million adults) with significant difficulties in functioning (10 facts on disability). This translates into nearly 15% of the world's population living with a disability. According to the WHO (n.d.), the numbers are rising.

Some of these limitations are permanent, while others are temporary. Some are relatively minor or so ubiquitous as to be a regularly accepted part of our species. Eyeglasses, hearing aids, balm for muscle sprains, arch supports, allergy medicine, and advice for depression, anxiety, or drinking problems fill our drugstore advertisements, blogs, and books stores.

Whether someone is on crutches following a fall on the ice, born with an intellectual disability, paraplegic from a car accident, clinically obese, alcoholic, chronically depressed, or nearsighted-temporary or permanent-major or minor impairment requires an adjustment. Adaptation to a greater or lesser extent to one's life circumstances is necessary for coping. Yet some adapt better than others, and some may even thrive following a physical or emotional challenge. Still, others do not, or cannot, adjust. What makes the difference? Is it a personality feature? A mindset? A type of resilience? What emerges from studies on how we accommodate to difficult circumstances is twofold. First, there are a myriad of responses to events with the potential to cause a disability. People respond differently to similar difficult or traumatic conditions. Secondly, the degree to which one must modify their life to accommodate the situation is not dependent on the severity or permanency of the disabilities alone. It is the intersection between one's circumstance and response to the disability where the capacity to respond effectively—or not—resides. This is to say that it is not the degree of disability that will determine how someone responds. It is how someone responds that determines the extent of disability.

This is not to diminish the often catastrophic experiences causing physical or psychological disability. Rather it highlights the fact that how people respond is separate from the event or condition itself. To paraphrase William James, circumstance does not make me, rather it reveals me.

By way of illustration two, ten, or a thousand people with the same potentially disabling condition may not all respond similarly. What has happened is a separate phenomenon from a response to what has happened. Inquisitiveness, being caring, and self-control are all core features of human virtues beneath one's character strengths that weigh in on how well or poorly one copes (McGrath et al., 2018). These character strengths are either awakened or inhibited by hardship. We will deal better or worse with a disabling condition depending on if we rise to the occasion or pull back. As resilience researcher Norman Garmezy so eloquently put it: Do you succumb or do you surmount?

In theorizing the functions of character strengths, Niemiec (2020) offers three functions for opportunity/well-being (i.e., functions of priming, mindfulness, and appreciation) and three core functions for managing adversity (i.e., functions of buffering, reappraisal, and resilience). For the latter functions, character strengths can serve to prevent some problems from occurring, reappraise challenges that occur, and support people in bouncing back from the problem. There are multiple expressions for each function and seemingly unlimited ways by which each might be expressed.

What an individual brings to the situation is not a static set of coping mechanisms, resilience strategies, or virtues, but rather an assortment of potentialities. The 24 character strengths can be ignited optimally, overused or underused in response to challenging events (Niemiec, 2019). In addition to this range of responses of how character strengths are revealed, limited, or unchanged by a potentially disabling condition, there is also the question of which strengths prepare us best.

This intersection of potentialities is most acutely evident and critical when a reaction to trauma has occurred, been averted—or transcended. Indeed, trauma and resilience researcher George Bonanno has offered the term Potentially Traumatic Event (PTE) to explain the wide capacity of responses possible to traumatic experiences (Bonanno, 2004). Some individuals after a PTE experience post-traumatic stress disorder (PTSD), a disabling condition with symptoms of depression and anxiety (Bonanno, 2021a, b). In the United States, about 90% of the population have experienced trauma (Kilpatrick, et al., 2013), while the lifetime prevalence of PTSD falls between 6% and 8% (Kessler, 1995). Others experiencing the same PTE have a life-changing reaction known as post-traumatic growth (PTG) (Tedeschi & Calhoun, 2004).

Individuals who experience PTG emerge from the event positively transformed including having better relationships, more responsivity to new possibilities, greater appreciation of life, and even higher levels of spiritual development. The variations of vulnerability (like PTSD) or vitality (PTG) that can emerge from a potentially traumatic event are broad. Researchers studying the intersection between the event and the individual see the inflection point as an influence on psychological resources responding to the trauma. They ask—how does trauma change us? Yet another perspective tries to illuminate what precedes this intersection. What prepares us best for hardship? The first highlights what happens after a trauma—the second investigates what happens before. This distinction is important because research on a post-traumatic event does not reveal who was better prepared. Furthermore, following a traumatic event a person who becomes disabled is often misjudged as having a lower quality of life by others who have not been affected. (Ubel et al., 2003).

The Resilience and Disability Paradoxes

Bonanno has long promoted the position that people are much more robust, more resilient, and less fragile than we think. He defines resilience as: "…the ability of individuals exposed to a potentially highly disruptive event to maintain both healthy psychological and physical functioning and the capacity for positive emotions" (Bonanno, 2004, p. 20). Resilience research typically shows correlation *after* the trauma, meaning we know who *became* resilient and in what way following a potentially traumatic event. However, this does not translate into understanding who will be resilient at an individual level when a disruptive event happens. This is known as the resilience paradox (Bonanno, 2021a, b). The focus is less on who becomes resilient and more on who has and how.

There is also a disability paradox (Albrecht & Devlieger, 1999). This paradox refers to how people with serious and persistent disabilities tend to report a good or excellent quality of life, yet professional evaluations of people with disabilities assume it is much lower than people with disability rate themselves. This discrepancy between quality-of-life estimates from patients and the public creates a gap between what people with disabilities actually experience and what an outside observer believes of their life satisfaction (Iezzoni et al., 2021).

However, this discrepancy is not limited to the general public. In a recent survey, over 82% of physicians believe people with disabilities have a lower quality of life. This shared prejudice has an impact on the disparities in healthcare services, including, but not limited to, access to screening, treatment, and communication for services (Iezzoni et al., 2021).

Part of the problem is that the general public and physicians engage in focalism (Wilson et al., 2000), or what has also been called diagnostic overshadowing (Molloy et al., 2021). The emphasis on one aspect of a disability eclipses other elements of well-being and functionality. The disability and the conditions around it are seen, but other strengths and qualities in the person's life may not be. This stigma is particularly true when it comes to individuals with intellectual and developmental disabilities and those with serious mental illnesses, including those reactions to trauma (Parekh & Childs, 2016).

These realities leave character strengths researchers with four broad questions surrounding reactions to traumatic events:

1. What happens after being exposed to a PTE?
2. What features were present before a PTE that predict how an individual might respond?
3. How does the person judge the quality of their life following the PTE?
4. If disabled, how are they judged by others?

The Science

Post-traumatic growth (PTG) is typically measured based on the degree to which an individual believes he or she has grown and developed as a result of struggling with trauma or crisis, whereas resilience is often thought of as a return to, or maintenance of, a baseline. As both have to do with reactions to disruptive events it might be more efficacious to see resilience as bouncing back and PTG as bouncing forward. Resilience is restorative and PTG is regenerative. How character strengths either facilitate or become different as a result of these processes has been a central part of understanding character strength development from the beginning.

One of the first studies to look at the connection between character strengths and trauma was conducted by Peterson and Seligman (2003) following the 911 terrorist attack in New York City. In this study VIA character strength scores before September 11 and 2 months after were compared for 4817 respondents revealing that seven strengths—gratitude, hope, love, kindness, leadership, spirituality, and teamwork—had increased. Ten months afterward these same strengths remained elevated—but to a lesser degree.

In another study, researchers investigated how multiple exposure to traumatic events in life might be correlated with higher character strength scores (Peterson et al., 2008). They asked about exposure to life-threatening accidents, natural or human disasters, physical attacks, sexual abuse, seeing someone killed, or being kidnapped. Of the 1739 individuals sampled, 25% reported one event, 18% reported two events, 9% reported three events, and 5% reported four or more. They found that exposure to greater experiences of trauma (one, two, three, or four or more) was correlated with higher character strengths. The more events people reported, the higher character strengths scores were—particularly those indicative of post-traumatic growth. In this study, several of the character strengths were assessing the very features Tedeschi and Calhoun (2004) contend happen during PTG such as kindness and love, demonstrating improved relationships, and openness to new possibilities, which were reflected in the strengths of curiosity, creativity, and love of learning. Additionally, greater appreciation of life was identified through appreciation of beauty, gratitude, zest, and higher levels of spiritual development reflected through one's spirituality score. In other words, the VIA Survey measurement tool helped to reflect if PTG had happened. The study found that while there was a direct linear relationship between the number of traumatic events experienced and increased character strength scores, the measures of gratitude, hope, and love did not follow this trend.

In a more broad study examining different kinds of adversities (victimization, stressful life events, and financial stress), the combination of strengths and adversities accounted for 58% of the variance in well-being, 50% of the variance in post-traumatic growth, and 50% of the variance in trauma symptoms (Hamby et al., 2018).

Taken together these studies support the adage from Friedrich Nietzsche's—*that which does not kill us makes us stronger*—by highlighting that certain character strengths are elevated following a single traumatic event, and multiple traumatic events might cause a similar phenomenon. These are demonstrations of important connections between character strengths and post-traumatic growth.

Yet, there is a curious difference in these findings. In response to 9/11, the seven character strengths found to improve following exposure to the event—gratitude, hope, kindness, leadership, love, spirituality, and teamwork—make intuitive sense and had increased. Yet in measuring responses to multiple trauma, three of the seven found to improve from the first study—gratitude, hope, and love specifically—had not been affected. Our response to highly disruptive events may elevate our character strengths, but which ones shift may be a more individualistic response.

To illustrate, a 2015 study (Schueller et al., 2015) followed pre- and post-character strength survey results for individuals within 100 miles surrounding large-scale gun violence occurring at Virginia Tech, Sandy Hook elementary school in Newtown, Connecticut, and an Aurora, Colorado, movie theater. The results were anything but consistent. For the Sandy Hook tragedy there were lower values for character strengths a month following, but higher values 2 months later. The reverse was true for the Virginia Tech trauma, and in the Aurora, Colorado, shooting no pattern emerged.

On the other side of the resilience paradox is the question of who becomes more resilient. Newer research has identified the correlation between character strengths and predicting greater resilience. In one study (Martinez-Marti & Ruch, 2017), all the strengths but spirituality correlated with resilience suggesting that higher character strength scores indicate higher resilience through greater energy, creativity, and flexibility. Indeed, in this study, it was hope, zest, and bravery that had the strongest correlation to resilience.

The Practice

From an applications perspective, a flexible mindset is an important area for exploration. Using Bonanno's framework, the energy, creativity, and flexibility accessed through elevated character strengths may be facilitating resilience and self-regulation through a flexible mindset (Bonanno, 2021a, b). A flexible mindset develops when one can reflect on the answers to four essential questions during a difficult time: What is happening? What do I need to do? What am I able to do? Is it working? Because we have an observer awareness as part of our human consciousness, we can learn to pause for thought as resilient people do when a crisis is upon us. This moment is when—and where—flexible thinking can be advanced. The ongoing assessment is where flexibility is nurtured. If the action chosen is working, then it becomes monitored. If not, then the mind begins cycling through the questions again. Like when we take a yoga class or do stretching exercises to develop our physical flexibility, there are ways to build a flexible mind. If you have ever woken up achy or felt a cramped muscle and felt the need to stretch, the discomfort prompts the need for relief through more flexibility. Once we see some relief, we may begin stretching as a regular part of our routine to prevent, not just cope with, the aches and pains. This is also true with emotional well-being.

The need for a flexible mindset is initially brought on by discomfort—or what we now know is disequilibrium. We need to stretch our minds when faced with an achy situation. Then, we learn to stretch to avoid aches. We better our resilience in disruptive situations by developing the ability to be flexible. We have learned from resilient people that this is what they do—and it is teachable.

The study and application of character strengths has arguably become one of the most important advances in the science of psychology, with rippling effects in education, psychotherapy, medicine, rehabilitation, business, and other fields (Mayerson, 2020). The broad and dynamic impact in its predictive capacity for well-being combined with its unique foundation in virtues offers a conceptually different way of understanding the human condition. Which of the character strengths to use as gateways to understanding reactions to trauma is likely to continually evolve based on synergies between science and practice. Ultimately, there may be many doors to one room where higher well-being and even thriving in response to trauma reside. With character strengths, there are 24 specific doors. Each with its own unique doorknob.

Of the 24 character strengths, it is the character strength of hope that offers a practical inflection point in response to a disruptive event causing a disability. When we talk about hope, we are referring to a belief that a positive future outcome is possible, combined with a desire for that outcome (Luo et al., 2020). Hope is the only character strength that requires negativity or uncertainty to be activated (Tomasulo, 2020). This makes hope a unique character strength as it requires a disruptive component to be provoked. The research suggests that hope both facilitates resilience and protects against PTSD as a meta-analysis showed greater hope is associated with lower levels of PTSD (Gallagher et al., 2020).

It has also been identified as one of the strengths that may both facilitate resilience by protecting against depression and impairment—and increase following a disruptive loss (Blanchard et al., 2021). Additionally, while hope and resilience together are distinct predictors of psychological flourishing for adult childhood trauma survivors, having hope and a hopeful mindset alone was a better predictor (Munoz et al., 2020).

More specifically, a lack of hope among older Japanese adults 7 months prior to the 2011 earthquake/tsunami were more likely to develop PTSD and depression 2.5 years after the disaster (Gero et al., 2021). Alternately, during resettlement, Kosovar war refugees with hope had a better chance of having post-traumatic growth and lower PTSD severity 10 months later (Ai et al., 2007). Similarly, police officials' PTEs encountered during the Global War on Terror experienced both less PTSD and greater PTG.

Having hope may offer these protective and regenerative effects because it assists the progress of more comprehensive positive outcomes beyond preventing PTSD. As an example, hope predicts less burnout, greater resilience, and lower secondary traumatization among healthcare workers (Ho & Lo, 2011; Passmore et al., 2020; Zanatta et al., 2020). It has also been associated with higher levels of forgiveness, empathy, and lower degrees of resentment (Nateghian et al., 2015).

It seems from the growing literature that hope has influence both before and after a PTE. Hope may be an essential character strength on both sides of trauma as it is indicative of protective and recovery features, reflecting, perhaps, who can access a flexible mindset. In light of this, the cultivation of hope and development of hope interventions may be the most direct way to use this transcendent strength. Hope appears to contribute to the common mechanism of recovery from PTSD. Because it is transdiagnostic, it can facilitate improvement across treatment modalities and, as it were, on both sides of the couch.

Hope can help patients with PTSD cope and achieve treatment goals (Snyder, 2002), experience greater connection to the therapist, less avoidant attachment, greater session frequency (Schiff & Levit, 2010), and have lower dropout rates (Semmlinger & Ehring, 2022). Yet, what may be the most surprising finding is that therapist's hope for their client may be a highly influential factor in treatment outcome (Bartholomew et al., 2019).

Hope increases as the result of various treatments for PTSD, such as Cognitive Processing Therapy (CPT), Prolonged Exposure, and Acceptance and Commitment Therapy (ACT) delivered in a naturalistic exposure-based treatment setting (Long,

2022). This means that hope may be a targeted factor that results as a facilitative byproduct in various treatment protocols. It may also be cultivated as a standalone intervention that has a direct influence on alleviating trauma (Kwon et al., 2015).

Perhaps the best of both worlds may be in combining the specific use of hope interventions with a treatment framework, such as positive psychotherapy (Rashid, 2020). As an example, this approach has been shown to be effective in eliciting post-traumatic growth in adults who have a brain injury (Karagiorgou et al., 2018).

Case Example

When looking at the swarms of research and meta-analyses it is important to refocus on the person-to-person features of having a framework, delivering the interventions, and following up and maintaining the transformation. It is the initial shattered assumption and feeling of a lack of empowerment, a type of hopelessness that follows a disruptive event that can make it traumatic. The clinician does not make an instant assessment, choose an intervention, and watch their patient transform. The process often begins with initial impressions, assessments, and understandings that need to be confirmed and understood, while an approach that emphasizes strengths and well-being is woven into the assessment. It is the frame of mind of the clinician that creates a foundation for change that allows for simultaneously lessening the suffering the client brings while highlighting the strengths that were and are being employed.

A character strength assessment gives the clinician the best opportunity to see the whole patient—not overshadow their perception through the aforementioned focalism or diagnostic overshadowing. Often by the time a patient arrives in the chair they have cultivated a narrative about what happened and their response, experienced changes in their social network, and had their daily life impacted to a greater or lesser degree. The goal initially is to hold and make the initial space safe for the patient to reveal their world post-trauma, yet for the clinician to hear the strengths embedded in the story of suffering. That is a key. Trauma clinicians often are over-focused on the details of the suffering while not paying attention to strengths that are present.

Jason, a 36-year-old man, was 5 years sober. He sought treatment for the traumatic event that initiated his sobriety. Drunk after midnight one night, he and his drinking buddy decide to swim around Manhattan. They strip and jump into the cold November waters of the Hudson River. Fifteen minutes into the attempt his friend is in trouble and goes under. Jason dives down repeatedly and on one attempt gets to his friend's body but is unable to bring him to the surface. After several failed efforts Jason is exhausted and needs to save himself. He swims to shore but in the struggle to pull himself out of the water he slips, falls, and goes unconscious. He wakes up to EMT, New York City Police, and The New York State Police Underwater Recovery Team. His friend has drowned, and the following day becomes his sobriety anniversary date. The wake, funeral, and investigation that followed were emotionally brutalizing, and within 6 months of the trauma he moved to North Carolina. In returning to the area for work he sought out therapy, and up to that point he had only used Alcoholics Anonymous for his recovery.

In an initial assessment for PTSD, he met the necessary criteria of having direct exposure, intrusive memories, flashbacks, and nightmares, and avoiding anything that would remind him of that night. Jason also experienced tremendous self-blame, isolation, and great difficulty having positive emotions. On and off he experienced all or some combination of these symptoms over the past 5 years.

At the same time as the PTSD assessment, his character strengths were surveyed. His top strengths were creativity, curiosity, honesty, judgment, and social intelligence. At the bottom were hope (#23) and self-regulation (#24).

While the course of his treatment will be discussed there will be a much greater emphasis on the initial stages. The practitioner's view of the patient and the patient's view of themselves become strengths-based rather than deficit-based. The goal of the therapist at this time is to use the strengths of character as tools to help the patient come into conflict with themselves and their narrative of how they see themselves. This is a nuanced form of cognitive restructuring designed to amplify character strengths that were and are being used as coping.

When Jason explained the details of the event and the aftermath. The feedback involved identifying a host of character strengths. Hearing Jason's story through the prism of character strengths allows the therapist to cognitively restructure the trauma-focused thoughts. To illustrate, some statements by the therapist included:

- *You've been sober for 5 years, and that could not have been easy.* (Self-regulation.)
- *It took a lot of courage to go and talk with your friend's family about what happened.* (Bravery.)
- *It sounds like the next day you made a decision to change the path you were on.* (Hope.)
- *You were honest with yourself about your drinking.* (Honesty.)
- *Admitting you were powerless allowed you to believe a high power could help you.* (Spirituality.)
- *You've made a lot of good connections in the AA community.* (Social intelligence.)
- *You've helped a lot of people.* (Love.)

The feedback from the therapist is designed to highlight that in addition to the symptoms of the trauma there are a wide number of coping mechanisms alongside them. There are also times when the therapist can invite a positive deviant—a time when this overuse or underuse of a strength is obvious and ask when something different (and better) may have happened.

- *It sounds like you put yourself down a lot.* (An overuse of Humility.) *Is there a time or a person you admire for how they handled a compliment?*
- *From what you are saying, except for AA meetings, you spend a lot of time alone and often feel lonely.* (An underuse of Love.) *Are there times other than meetings that you also enjoy connecting, or are even intimate with people?*

The initial, foundational meetings introduced the idea that strengths and struggles coexist.

For Jason and true for many people who experience trauma, there are numerous insights and practices that come together to foster healing. The opposites of pain and growth, limits and expansion, self-reliance and needing support, are mixed in with the process of healing and coping (Captari et al., 2021). The recognition of these paradoxes are collectively known as post-traumatic depreciation (PTD) (Taku et al. 2021). Along with the good comes the bad, and vice versa. To cope with these polarities, trauma survivors with PTG use dialectical thinking (Tedeschi & Calhoun, 2004). Dialectical thinking is when two polar opposite thoughts (like vulnerability and strength) are held together in awareness. This is a central feature in the findings about PTG and the literature on the relationship between wisdom and subjective well-being (Zacher & Staudinger, 2018). While the events of a difficult reaction are not desirable, there is goodness and growth that can come from having to face them (Tedeschi & Calhoun, 2004).

This is the spirit of the intervention behind amplifying character strengths in the face of a traumatic narrative. This can help loosen the grip of intrusive ruminative thinking.

While the initial stages of this are highlighted here, there is the necessity of ongoing practice. This includes specific techniques and skills and strategies for reducing stress (e.g., Mindfulness Based Stress Reduction, Grossman et al., 2004), becoming more mindful of character strengths (Niemiec, 2023), meeting others and learning interpersonal skills (Group therapy, Yalom & Leszcz, 2020), cultivating a gratitude habit (Wood et al., 2010), and developing a personal loving-kindness meditation practice (Fredrickson et al., 2008). These help to lead individuals like Jason to a successful therapeutic outcome.

The foundation of character strength acknowledgment, fostering dialectical thinking for the purpose of post-traumatic depreciation, and then adding specific emotional self-regulation and interpersonal skills helped Jason become hopeful and whole. Ultimately after about a year and a half of therapy, he was promoted to supervisor where he worked because of his technical and interpersonal skills and got engaged. It was not lost on Jason that his appreciation of beauty and excellence, and his social intelligence, had gotten him the promotion at work, and the engagement allowed him to make a commitment to intimacy.

In retaking the VIA Survey as he exited therapy, the character strength that made the greatest change was that of hope. It went from #23 to #8.

Future Directions

There is far more unknown than known in the understanding and integration of character strengths and trauma. While some interesting findings have emerged, there has been inconsistency. Future research will examine individual and contextual differences in character strengths across different types and degrees of trauma.

Within the resilience paradox particularly, further understanding is needed for those character strengths that support greater resilience. Will the research connecting zest, hope, and bravery with greater resilience (Martinez-Marti & Ruch, 2017) be replicated? What is the role of delving into and expressing one's most authentic qualities—signature strengths? Perhaps the loss of self that can occur in many traumatic incidents can be recovered by maintaining strength with one's most core qualities? How might character strengths enable or inhibit a resilient response to trauma? The balance and imbalance of character strengths as reflected by overuse, underuse, and optimal-use (Niemiec, 2019) has not received attention in cases of trauma and is also an area ripe for potential for scientists and practitioners.

Key Takeaways

- It is not the degree of disability that will determine how someone responds. It is how someone responds that determines the extent of disability.
- Potentially Traumatic Event (PTE) is used to explain the wide capacity of responses possible to traumatic experiences.
- Individuals who experience post-traumatic growth (PTG) emerge from the event positively impacted and in some cases transformed including having better relationships, more responsivity to new possibilities, greater appreciation of life, and even higher levels of spiritual development.
- Researchers studying the intersection between the event and the individual see the inflection point as an influence on psychological resources responding to the trauma. Research on a post-traumatic event does not reveal who was better prepared.
- Resilience research typically shows correlation *after* the trauma, meaning we know who *became* resilient and in what way following a potentially traumatic event. However, this does not translate into understanding who will be resilient at an individual level when a disruptive event happens. This is known as the resilience paradox. The focus is less on who becomes resilient and more on who has and how.
- There is also a disability paradox. In this paradox people with serious and persistent disabilities report a good or excellent quality of life. Yet non-disabled evaluations of people with disabilities assume it is much lower than people with disability rate themselves. This discrepancy between quality-of-life estimates from patients and the public creates a gap between what people with disabilities actually experience and what an outside observer believes of their life satisfaction.
- Resilience can be seen as bouncing back and PTG as bouncing forward. Resilience is restorative and PTG is regenerative.
- Our response to highly disruptive events may elevate our character strengths, but which ones shift may be a more individualistic response.

(continued)

- The energy, creativity, and flexibility accessed through elevated character strengths may be facilitating resilience and self-regulation through a flexible mindset. A flexible mindset develops when one can reflect on the answers to four essential questions during a difficult time: What is happening? What do I need to do? What am I able to do? Is it working?
- Hope is the only character strength that requires negativity or uncertainty to be activated. This makes hope a unique character strength as it requires a disruptive component to be provoked. The research suggests that hope both facilitates resilience and protects against PTSD; a meta-analysis showed greater hope is associated with lower levels of PTSD. It has also been identified as one of the strengths that may both facilitate resilience by protecting against depression and impairment and increase following a disruptive loss.
- Hope appears to contribute to the common mechanism of recovery from PTSD. Because it is transdiagnostic it can facilitate improvement across treatment modalities and, as it were, on both sides of the couch.
- The opposites of pain and growth, limits and expansion, self-reliance and needing support are mixed in with the process of healing and coping. The recognition of these paradoxes is collectively known as post-traumatic depreciation (PTD). Along with the good comes the bad, and vice versa.
- To cope with these polarities, trauma survivors with PTG use dialectical thinking. Dialectical thinking occurs when two polar opposite thoughts (like vulnerability and strength) are held together in awareness. This is a central feature in the findings about PTG and the literature on the relationship between wisdom and subjective well-being.
- While the events of a difficult reaction are not desirable, there is goodness and growth that can come from having to face them.

References

Ai, A. L., Tice, T. N., Whitsett, D. D., Ishisaka, T., & Chim, M. (2007). Posttraumatic symptoms and growth of Kosovar war refugees: The influence of hope and cognitive coping. *The Journal of Positive Psychology, 2*, 55–65. https://doi.org/10.1080/17439760601069341

Albrecht, G. L., & Devlieger, P. J. (1999). The disability paradox: High quality of life against all odds. *Social Science & Medicine, 48*(8), 977–988. https://doi.org/10.1016/s0277-9536(98)00411-0

Bartholomew, T. T., Gundel, B. E., Li, H., Joy, E. E., Kang, E., & Scheel, M. J. (2019). The meaning of therapists' hope for their clients: A phenomenological study. *Journal of Counseling Psychology, 66*(4), 496.

Blanchard, T., McGrath, R. E., & Jayawickreme, E. (2021). Resilience in the face of interpersonal loss: The role of character strengths. *Applied Psychology: Health and Well-Being, 13*(4), 817–834.

Bonanno, G. A. (2004). Loss, trauma, and human resilience: have we underestimated the human capacity to thrive after extremely aversive events? *American Psychologist, 59*(1), 20.

Bonanno, G. A. (2021a). *The end of trauma: How the new science of resilience changes how we think about PTSD*. Basic Books.

Bonanno, G. A. (2021b). The resilience paradox. *European Journal of Psychotraumatology, 12*(1), 1942642.

Captari, L. E., Riggs, S. A., & Stephen, K. (2021). Attachment processes following traumatic loss: A mediation model examining identity distress, shattered assumptions, prolonged grief, and posttraumatic growth. *Psychological Trauma: Theory, Research, Practice, and Policy, 13*(1), 94.

Fredrickson, B. L., Cohn, M. A., Coffey, K. A., Pek, J., & Finkel, S. M. (2008). Open hearts build lives: positive emotions, induced through loving-kindness meditation, build consequential personal resources. *Journal of Personality and Social Psychology, 95*(5), 1045.

Gallagher, M. W., Long, L. J., & Phillips, C. A. (2020). Hope, optimism, self-efficacy, and post-traumatic stress disorder: A meta-analytic review of the protective effects of positive expectancies. *Journal of Clinical Psychology, 76*(3), 329–355.

Gero, K., Aida, J., Shirai, K., Kondo, K., & Kawachi, I. (2021). Dispositional optimism and disaster resilience: A natural experiment from the 2011 Great East Japan Earthquake and Tsunami. *Social Science & Medicine, 273*, 113777. https://doi.org/10.1016/j.socscimed.2021.113777

Grossman, P., Niemann, L., Schmidt, S., & Walach, H. (2004). Mindfulness-based stress reduction and health benefits: A meta-analysis. *Journal of Psychosomatic Research, 57*(1), 35–43.

Hamby, S., Grych, J., & Banyard, V. (2018). Resilience portfolios and poly-strengths: Identifying protective factors associated with thriving after adversity. *Psychology of Violence, 8*(2), 172–183. https://doi.org/10.1037/vio0000135

Ho, S. M. Y., & Lo, R. S. Y. (2011). Dispositional hope as a protective factor among medical emergency professionals: A preliminary investigation. *Traumatology, 17*, 3–9. https://doi.org/10.1177/1534765611426786

Iezzoni, L. I., Rao, S. R., Ressalam, J., Bolcic-Jankovic, D., Agaronnik, N. D., Donelan, K., et al. (2021). Physicians' perceptions of people with disability and their health care: Study reports the results of a survey of physicians' perceptions of people with disability. *Health Affairs, 40*(2), 297–306.

Karagiorgou, O., Evans, J. J., & Cullen, B. (2018). Post-traumatic growth in adult survivors of brain injury: A qualitative study of participants completing a pilot trial of brief positive psychotherapy. *Disability and Rehabilitation, 40*(6), 655–659.

Kessler, R. C. (1995). Posttraumatic stress disorder in the national comorbidity survey. *Archives of General Psychiatry, 52*, 1048. https://doi.org/10.1001/archpsyc.1995.03950240066012

Kilpatrick, D. G., Resnick, H. S., Milanak, M. E., Miller, M. W., Keyes, K. M., & Friedman, M. J. (2013). National estimates of exposure to traumatic events and PTSD prevalence using *DSM-IV* and *DSM-5* criteria: *DSM-5* PTSD prevalence. *Journal of Traumatic Stress, 26*, 537–547. https://doi.org/10.1002/jts.21848

Kwon, P., Birrueta, M., Faust, E., & Brown, E. R. (2015). The role of hope in preventive interventions. *Social and Personality Psychology Compass, 9*(12), 696–704.

Long, L. J. (2022). Hope and PTSD. *Current Opinion in Psychology, 48*, 101472. https://doi.org/10.1016/j.copsyc.2022.101472

Luo, S. X., Van Horen, F., Millet, K., & Zeelenberg, M. (2020). What we talk about when we talk about hope: A prototype analysis. *Emotion, 22*(4), 751–768. https://doi.org/10.1037/emo0000821

Martínez-Martí, M. L., & Ruch, W. (2017). Character strengths predict resilience over and above positive affect, self-efficacy, optimism, social support, self-esteem, and life satisfaction. *The Journal of Positive Psychology, 12*(2), 110–119. https://doi.org/10.1080/17439760.2016.1163403

Mayerson, N. H. (2020). The character strengths response: an urgent call to action. *Frontiers in Psychology, 11*, 2106.

McGrath, R., Greenberg, M., & Hall-Simmonds, A. (2018). Scarecrow, Tin Woodsman, and Cowardly Lion: The three factor model of virtue. *Journal of Positive Psychology, 13*(4), 373–392. https://doi.org/10.1080/17439760.2017.1326518

Molloy, R., Brand, G., Munro, I., & Pope, N. (2021). Seeing the complete picture: A systematic review of mental health consumer and health professional experiences of diagnostic overshadowing. *Journal of Clinical Nursing, 32*, 1662. https://doi.org/10.1111/jocn.16151

Munoz, R. T., Hanks, H., & Hellman, C. M. (2020). Hope and resilience as distinct contributors to psychological flourishing among childhood trauma survivors. *Traumatology, 26*(2), 177.

Nateghian, S., Dastgiri, S. S., & Mullet, E. (2015). Dispositional forgiveness and PTSD among Iranian veterans of the 1980–1988 war. *Journal of Loss and Trauma, 20*, 123–130. https://doi.org/10.1080/15325024.2013.831262

Niemiec, R. M. (2019). Finding the golden mean: the overuse, underuse, and optimal use of character strengths. *Counselling Psychology Quarterly, 32*(3–4), 453–471.

Niemiec, R. M. (2020). Six functions of character strengths for thriving at times of adversity and opportunity: A theoretical perspective. *Applied Research in Quality of Life, 15*, 551–572. https://doi.org/10.1007/s11482-018-9692-2

Niemiec, R. M. (2023). *Mindfulness and character strengths: A practitioner's guide to MBSP* (2nd ed.). Hogrefe.

Parekh, R., & Childs, E. W. (Eds.). (2016). *Stigma and prejudice: Touchstones in understanding diversity in healthcare*. Springer.

Passmore, S., Hemming, E., McIntosh, H. C., & Hellman, C. M. (2020). The relationship between hope, meaning in work, secondary traumatic stress, and burnout among child abuse pediatric clinicians. *TPJ, 24*(19), 087. https://doi.org/10.7812/TPP/19.087

Peterson, C., & Seligman, M. E. (2003). Character strengths before and after September 11. *Psychological Science, 14*(4), 381–384.

Peterson, C., Park, N., Pole, N., D'Andrea, W., & Seligman, M. E. (2008). Strengths of character and posttraumatic growth. *Journal of Traumatic Stress, 21*(2), 214–217.

Rashid, T. (2020). Positive psychotherapy. In F. Maggino (Ed.), *Encyclopedia of quality of life and well-being research*. Springer. https://doi.org/10.1007/978-3-319-69909-7_3378-2

Schiff, M., & Levit, S. (2010). Correlates of therapeutic alliance and treatment outcomes among Israeli female methadone patients. *Research on Social Work Practice, 20*, 380–390. https://doi.org/10.1177/1049731509347854

Schueller, S. M., Jayawickreme, E., Blackie, L. E., Forgeard, M. J., & Roepke, A. M. (2015). Finding character strengths through loss: An extension of Peterson and Seligman (2003). *The Journal of Positive Psychology, 10*(1), 53–63.

Semmlinger, V., & Ehring, T. (2022). Predicting and preventing dropout in research, assessment and treatment with refugees. *Clin Psychology and Psychoth, 29*, 767–782. https://doi.org/10.1002/cpp.2672

Snyder, C. R. (2002). Hope theory: Rainbows in the mind. *Psychological Inquiry, 13*, 249–275. https://doi.org/10.1207/S15327965PLI1304_01

Sussex Publishers. (n.d.). *The disability paradox*. Psychology Today. Retrieved March 6, 2023. Found at https://www.psychologytoday.com/us/blog/disability-is-diversity/202209/the-disability-paradox

Taku, K., Tedeschi, R. G., Shakespeare-Finch, J., Krosch, D., David, G., et al. (2021). Posttraumatic growth (PTG) and posttraumatic depreciation (PTD) across ten countries: Global validation of the PTG-PTD theoretical model. *Personality and Individual Differences, 169*, 110222.

Tedeschi, R. G., & Calhoun, L. G. (2004). Posttraumatic growth: Conceptual foundations and empirical evidence. *Psychological Inquiry, 15*(1), 1–18.

Tomasulo, D. (2020). *Learned hopefulness: The power of positivity to overcome depression*. New Harbinger Publications.

Ubel, P. A., Loewenstein, G., & Jepson, C. (2003). Whose quality of life? A commentary exploring discrepancies between health state evaluations of patients and the general public. *Quality of Life Research, 12*, 599–607. https://doi.org/10.1023/A:1025119931010

Wilson, T. D., Wheatley, T., Meyers, J. M., Gilbert, D. T., & Axsom, D. (2000). Focalism: a source of durability bias in affective forecasting. *Journal of Personality and Social Psychology, 78*(5), 821.

Wood, A. M., Froh, J. J., & Geraghty, A. W. (2010). Gratitude and well-being: A review and theoretical integration. *Clinical Psychology Review, 30*(7), 890–905.

World Health Organization. (n.d.). *10 facts on disability*. World Health Organization. https://www.who.int/news-room/facts-in-pictures/detail/disabilities. Accessed on 6 Mar 2023.

Yalom, I. D., & Leszcz, M. (2020). *The theory and practice of group psychotherapy*. Basic books.

Zacher, H., & Staudinger, U. M. (2018). Wisdom and well-being. In *Handbook of well-being*. DEF Publishers.

Zanatta, F., Maffoni, M., & Giardini, A. (2020). Resilience in palliative healthcare professionals: A systematic review. *Support Care Cancer, 28*, 971–978. https://doi.org/10.1007/s00520-019-05194-1

Chapter 6
Psychiatric Disabilities and Character Strengths

We are not enemies, but friends. We must not be enemies. Though passion may have strained, it must not break our bonds of affection. The mystic chords of memory will swell when again touched, as surely they will be, by the better angels of our nature.

—Abraham Lincoln

The Concepts

The history of psychology's treatment of psychiatric disabilities has largely focused on alleviating suffering (Seligman & Csikszentmihalyi, 2000). This approach has resulted in research on interventions capable of decreasing the frequency and intensity of symptoms. Following validation of these approaches, training programs to teach these interventions and their widespread application became the norm. While admirable, this deficit-based approach has resulted in a *treatment-prevalence paradox* (TPP) (Ormel et al., 2022). This paradox explains that in spite of the vast array of treatments developed to cope with mental illness, the occurrence and severity continue to grow at a rate faster than the treatment's effectiveness.

Psychiatric disabilities can present many challenges and difficulties for those who experience them. Chief among the issues with debilitating mental illness is the chronicity of symptoms (Prince et al., 2007). Because mental health issues become problematic largely due to their persistence, a treatment should be layered in its approach. Ongoing mental health issues present a very different problem than transient emotional states. When someone's mental anguish has become their constant companion, they adjust to this persistent struggle in ways that present the difficulties as an identity. The disorder seeps into their psyche to become part of who they are. This is a vastly different experience than a passing, short-lived, emotional "episode" one might have. This episodic deviation is from a normally moderately

R. M. Niemiec, D. Tomasulo, *Character Strengths and Abilities Within Disabilities*, Positive Psychology and Disability Series,
https://doi.org/10.1007/978-3-031-36294-1_6

resilient and happy person. It has not become their identity. It is a contradiction to who they are. As such, realigning them to their norm is an adjustment, not a restructuring.

But when repetitive thoughts, behaviors, and emotions crowd out the less pathological experiences, the norm is what is not okay. What happens then is that the individual knows no other way to behave, think, or feel, and stops trying to manage the display. When this occurs, the good features of one's life sink below the pathology and becomes hidden from the individual themselves. The real problem with this situation is that it also remains hidden from the professional. Our assessment, treatment, and criteria by which we measure success gets hijacked by the disability, pathology, and sickness. Looking past someone's psychiatric disability rarely occurs, and if the positive elements in one's life are witnessed or acknowledged, the tools to cultivate it were traditionally missing.

Yet, to yield truly corrective experiences for individuals with chronic and persistent mental illness the symptoms and the assets need to be facilitated. Both downregulation of the negative symptoms and upregulation of well-being elements need to be employed (Rubin-Falcone et al., 2018).

Those working with individuals with psychiatric disabilities need to acknowledge the difficulties as well as the strengths they bring to the circumstance. Stigmatization is one of those barriers as several character strengths—self-regulation, perseverance, spirituality, and prudence (and to a lesser extent, hope and zest)—were associated with greater stigmatizing of people with mental illness in a large sample (Datu & Niemiec, 2023). Most of these are self-oriented character strengths that do not emphasize "the other." In contrast, the other-oriented strengths of kindness, fairness, and social intelligence were strongly associated with less stigmatizing of people with mental illness. An approach that shifts the script to see the humanness of the character strengths in people with mental illness—while perhaps playing into certain other-oriented character strengths of one's own—might be a more balanced and compassionate pathway forward.

Interventions will be most effective if triaged. Alleviating suffering will allow for upregulation to happen more readily. But, both the pain and potentiality need to be part of the assessment. Three guidelines for an assessment that includes strategies for down and up regulation simultaneously are given in the following text.

The first order of intervention should be to understand (as best as possible) the causes and then to reduce the negative features of one's symptoms. This will allow for some relief, but does not necessarily enhance, improve, or facilitate well-being. While the downregulating of negative emotions can have a therapeutic effect (De Witte et al., 2017; Eippert et al., 2007; Zaehringer et al., 2020), and the explicit and implicit suppression of an emotional response can be helpful (Katsumi & Dolcos, 2020), these downregulating interventions do not consistently yield a corresponding increase in positive emotions directly. Being in emotional pain does not make you happy or positive. It reduces suffering—which is a foundation and perhaps a springboard for improving well-being, but is not well-being itself. Not being anxious, depressed, psychotic, or rageful can be alleviating, but falls short of increasing joy, love, contentment, and gratitude. The implication is that strategies to decrease negative emotions may need to be incorporated with strategies designed to increase positive ones to effectively yield sustainable change.

Secondly, the goal then is to find ways to have these interventions produce sustainable changes, meaning that as the reduced suffering lasts, opportunities for well-being improve and evolve. It is the sustainability of non-pathological states that creates the conditions for improvement toward thriving—but as with well-being, is not thriving itself. These interventions need to be used to prevent relapse and promote prevention. If no interventions exist for the population to be served, evidence-informed interventions must be developed, and then tested for effectiveness.

Next, these separate interventions needed to upregulate positive emotions should have as their goal, tipping the scale in favor of thriving and flourishing. Yet most of the effort in psychological research prior to 2000 was aimed at the first objective—to downregulate negative consequences of symptoms (Seligman & Csikszentmihalyi, 2000). As a result, sustainability, relapse deterrence, and prevention strategies lagged, and the last set of needed positive interventions was almost completely absent from the research and applied sectors. This situation has changed and the emphasis on emotional regulation more often includes both downregulation of negative experiences and the upregulation of positivity. What has been missing is a framework for assessing both and developing treatment plans that administer both depending on the needs of the individual.

As an individual's emotional self-regulation is taking a more prominent role in treatment paradigms, the historically disproportionate emphasis on interventions to reduce suffering has evolved to accommodate and include interventions that increase positivity. This provides the individual with the capacity to self-regulate by striving toward a balance rather than trying to leverage emotional pain. There is now a dramatic shift to move toward a *broaden and build* way of shifting one's emotional experience to the positive (Fredrickson, 2004). The upregulating of positive emotions through specific strategies has created a class of investigations. These explorations demonstrate that investment in engagement of positive interventions leads to increased positive emotions. The result is a sustainable shift in feelings of subjective well-being. In general, upregulating positive emotions appears to reduce negative thoughts and affect (Chiesa et al., 2013; Livingstone & Srivastava, 2012; Quoidbach et al., 2015; Silton et al., 2020), as well as increase prosocial behavior (Iwamoto et al., 2020). Subsequent research looked more broadly at a myriad of areas in positive psychology (including character strengths) making the scientific argument that these areas buffer and bolster mental well-being (Waters et al., 2021). These findings mean that increasing positivity offers a lot to help make someone whole.

While the call to reshape the nature of treatment and research in psychology is barely 20 years old, the call for this shift dates back further. Medical sociology Professor Aaron Antonovsky (1979) coined the phrase "salutogenesis," which was an invitation for medical and psychological approaches to look beyond disease for treatment options—to rigorously search for factors and features that nurture and facilitate health and well-being. The functional implication of salutogenesis is that a treatment approach should encompass not only the reduction of distress and coping strategies, but also provide ways to add balance in the direction of emotional well-being.

Toward this end, a character strength approach is a salutogenetic framework. It allows for well-being to emerge as a regulation of perception refocusing on those attributes of an individual that offer whole-health flourishing. It does not dismiss, fail to notice, or minimize difficulties that carry an emotional weight. It is not blinded or overshadowed by them either. Rather than emphasizing sickness, pathology, and disability, character development turns attention toward possibilities rather than problems alone. It regulates and strengthens the perception of what can be done—not simply what cannot.

To exemplify this, we turn to the term, *eunoia*, from ancient Greece and used by Aristotle, which translates into a well mind and beautiful thinking. It is also a rarely used medical term specifically used to describe normal mental health. From the Greek eu (i.e., well, good) and noos (i.e., mind, spirit), it is interesting we have a term for good mental health and wellness we do not use, and most of us have never heard of. As an underused medical term its lack of use and familiarity may be because the medical model, on which psychology has been based, requires symptoms, syndromes, and illnesses to be engaged. In psychopathology, to be free from symptoms is assumed to be a return to a well mind, but if it is not understood what a well mind is, we are left with a reductionistic goal that simply has not worked as well as we would have hoped. Without knowing exactly what a well mind and normal mental health means, those looking to reduce the symptoms of a psychiatric disability are left with only one ill-fated goal. They operate under the inference that once the symptoms are gone normal mental health returns. This chapter pursues eunoia and the pursuit of mental health that can build up well-being while also reducing mental afflictions.

The Science

The Value of Strengths Buffering

The creation, accentuation, or bolstering of mental health with character strengths (in people with and without psychiatric problems) has received attention over the years. Character strengths have been shown to buffer against mental problems (Demirci et al., 2019; Huta & Hawley, 2010; Niemiec, 2020; Waters et al., 2021). In a sample of older adults, character strengths were associated with low levels of suicidal ideation representing a strong protective effect (Cheng et al., 2020), while in a study of 2000 Japanese adults, love and engagement were significant predictors of suicidal ideation indicating that building loving relationships and active engagement in the world might be important protective factors for suicide (Sueki, 2020). A study in the UK found strengths use moderated the relationship between paranoia and life satisfaction, while strengths use was positively associated with life satisfaction and positive self-beliefs (McTiernan et al., 2020).

The Dual Role of Strengths for Mental Health

Recently, Niemiec (2023) took a different approach to examine the dual role character strengths have in promoting mental well-being and in reducing symptoms and suffering. He asked over 12,000 individuals about their perception of the character strengths they used to create greater mental health (physical health, social health, and other areas were also examined), regardless of their mental health status. The character strengths that emerged strongest for mental health were love, kindness, curiosity, creativity, and perspective. This points to the value of both heart strengths and mind strengths for mental well-being. The strengths of love and kindness might manifest as a self-compassion (Neff, 2003) and in cultivating loving-kindness practices (Salzberg, 1995) involving warmth and care for oneself and others; the strengths of curiosity, creativity, and perspective are strengths of cognition and wisdom and involve the gathering and sharing of knowledge.

Niemiec (2023) also found that individuals had a distinct preference to use their character strengths for emotional coping at difficult times, such as using strengths to understand/face feelings or to manage feelings in a new or positive way (42% of respondents), as opposed to behavioral action (23%) or changes in thinking (25%). This finding dovetails with another finding in this research—those character strengths that participants wished they could use to improve their mental health. Four of the top five character strength *wishes* were self-regulation, bravery, perseverance, and forgiveness. Applied to emotional coping, the strength of bravery can help individuals face, confront, and name/label their feelings, perseverance to stay with the feeling, self-regulation to manage or control feelings, and forgiveness to let them go.

Overuse, Underuse, and Optimal-Use of Strengths

As we have argued, the absence of deficits alone cannot be the goal of well-being. Rather, the cultivation of optimal use of character strengths needs to be installed as a primary means of reducing psychopathology. Toward this goal there are two foundational premises. The first is that learning to thrive reduces suffering. Second, only lowering misery invites its return.

The shift toward this way of thinking involves cultivating a dialectical way of thinking where dealing with challenges and life's obstacles are balanced with seizing and creating opportunities for growth. Life's challenges are a good starting point for understanding how effective character strengths can be used in coping. Strengths in this manner become as real or as important as symptoms and disorders (Rashid, 2015).

An initial attempt at applying character strengths to psychotherapy was offered by Peterson (2006) noting "disorders" of character and he framed these as exaggeration, absence, and opposite of several character strengths. For example, for the strength of bravery, he described the exaggeration as foolhardiness, its absence as fright, and its opposite as cowardice. Seligman (2015) added that thinking in this way might have advantages over the DSM categorization, such as, systematically relating to one another (instead of a laundry list of disorders); defined by universality thus lending to cross-cultural psychopathology; being purer, natural classes; not tied to a medical model demanding symptoms, syndrome, and illness; and not reductionistic demanding a biological basis as the ultimate criterion.

Unfortunately, in testing this framework with a variety of practitioners, educators, and scholars across the globe, this model fell flat, repeatedly, from practical and conceptual perspectives, often leading practitioners feeling the approach was too erudite, complex, and confusing. But it was used as the foundation for important revisions. A new model was developed to be more conceptually clean, straightforward to study, philosophically and theoretically aligned, and accessible for scientists. This new model, the overuse, underuse, and optimal-use of character strengths, by Niemiec (2014) offered an echoing back to concepts of Aristotle (fourth BCE/2000) such as balance, a strength as having two opposites, and a contextual golden mean for expression. It explained that each of the 24 character strengths was on a continuum of more or less—too much or too little—and the center was the optimal strengths use or the golden mean, referring to the right combination of character strength expressed to the right degree in the right situation. For example, the underuse of curiosity is boredom and apathy, the optimal-use is being an explorer, open to novelty, while the overuse is being nosy and intrusive. In contrast, the underuse of leadership is being particularly passive and over-compliant, the optimal-use is positively influencing others, and the overuse is being controlling and authoritarian. If someone was high in kindness and helps people who do not want or need help, that is overuse, while being inattentive or uncaring to those in need is an underuse in that situation. To exemplify this, an individual walking around the city who ties the shoelaces of each person they meet will be perceived by many as being intrusive with the attempted kindness, while the person who intentionally looks away and ignores the elderly woman struggling to get on the train with her luggage would be showing an indifference or an underuse of kindness.

Niemiec (2019) updated the model and offered a mapping of hypothetical dimensions of overuse and underuse for each character strength along with short descriptions of optimal-use. As a general rule of thumb, in order to qualify as strengths overuse or underuse, the character strength must be causing sub-optimal functioning or a negative impact of some kind upon oneself or others. As a parallel, the internal distress of an Axis I disorder would align with negative impact on oneself while Axis II disorders might align with negative impact on others (as well as oneself). Table 6.1 shows the updated language for overuse, underuse, and optimal-use.

These revisions by Niemiec were meant to apply to any person's inner experiences, life challenges, suffering, or context, not limited to nor excluding those with psychopathology. The model has been discussed in the context of psychopathology and mental disorders from a theoretical perspective (Rashid & Seligman, 2018). In addition, the character strengths have been discussed as moderators of clinical

Table 6.1 Character strengths dimensions of overuse, underuse, and optimal-use, adapted from Niemiec (2019)

Character strength	Underuse	Overuse	Optimal-use
Creativity	Conforming; plain/dull; unimaginative	Eccentric; odd; scattered	Uniqueness that is practical; original, clever, imaginative
Curiosity	Bored; uninterested; apathetic; self-involved	Nosy; intrusive, self-serving	"Explorer," intrigued, open, novelty-seeker
Judgment	Illogical; naïve; unreflective; closed-minded	Narrow-minded; cynical; rigid; indecisive; lost in one's head	Seeing 360 degrees of details; analytical, detail oriented, open-minded, rational, logical
Love of learning	Smug; complacent with knowledge or growth; uninterested	Know-it-all; elitist; overwhelming	Going deep with knowledge; information-seeking; lifelong learner
Perspective	Shallow; superficial; lacking confidence	Overbearing; arrogant; disconnected	Sees and offers the wider review; wise; integrating viewpoints beyond one's own
Bravery	Cowardly; unwilling to act; unwilling to be vulnerable	Risk-taking; foolish; overconfident; unconcerned of others' reactions	Facing fears; confronting adversity; valor
Perseverance	Lazy; helpless; giving up	Stubborn; struggles to let go; fixated	Task completer; persistent and gritty; overcoming all obstacles
Honesty	Phony; dishonest; inauthentic; lacking integrity	Self-righteous; rude; inconsiderate	True to oneself, authentic to others; truth-sharer and seeker; sincere; without pretense
Zest	Sloth-like; passive; sedentary; tired	Hyper; overactive; annoying	Enthusiasm for life; happy; active; energized
Love	Isolating; cut-off from others; afraid to care; not relating	Emotional overkill; misaligned with others' needs; sugary sweet/touchy-feely	Genuine, reciprocal warmth; connected; relational fulfillment
Kindness	Indifferent; selfish; uncaring to yourself; mean-spirited	Compassion-fatigue; intrusive; overly focused on others	Doing for others; caring; compassionate; generous; nice and friendly
Social intelligence	Clueless; disconnected; socially naïve; emotionally insensitive	Over-analytical; self-deception; overly sensitive	Tuned in, then savvy; knowing what makes others tick; empathic; emotionally intelligent
Teamwork	Self-serving; individualistic; going it alone	Dependent; lost in groupthink; blind obedience; loss of individuality	Participative; contributing to group efforts; loyal; socially responsible; collaborative

(continued)

Table 6.1 (continued)

Character strength	Underuse	Overuse	Optimal-use
Fairness	Prejudice; partisanship; complacency	Detached; indecisive on justice issues; uncaring justice	Champions equal opportunity for all; care- and justice-based; moral concern
Leadership	Follower; compliant and mousy; passive	Bossy; controlling; authoritarian	Positively influencing others; organizing groups; leading around a vision
Forgiveness	Vengeful; merciless; easily triggered by others	Permissive; doormat; too lenient or soft	Letting go of hurt when wronged; giver of second changes; accepting shortcomings
Humility	Arrogant; braggadocio; self-focused; heavy ego needs	Self-deprecation; limited self-image; subservient; withholding about oneself	Clear view of oneself; focuses attention on others; sees own limitations; modest
Prudence	Reckless; thrill-seeking; acting before thinking	Stuffy; prudish; rigid; passive	Wisely cautious; thinks before speaks; planful; goal-oriented; risk-manager
Self-regulation	Self-indulgent; emotional dysregulation; impulsive; undisciplined; unfocused	Constricted; inhibited; tightly wound; obsessive	Self-manager of vices; mindful; disciplined
Appreciation of beauty and excellence	Oblivious; stuck in autopilot; mindlessness	Snobbery; perfectionistic; intolerant; unrelenting standards	Seeing the life behind things; awe/wonder in the presence of beauty; admiration for excellence; elevation for the goodness of others
Gratitude	Entitled; unappreciative; self-absorbed	Ingratiation; contrived; profuse; repetitive	Attitude of thankfulness; connected; appreciating positives
Hope	Negative; pessimistic; past-oriented; despair	Unrealistic; Pollyannaish; head in the clouds, blind optimism	Positive expectations; optimistic; confidence in goals and future
Humor	Overly serious; stilted/stiff; flat affect	Tasteless/offensive; giddy; socially inappropriate	Laughter/joy with others; seeing the lighter side; playful
Spirituality	Lack of purpose or meaning in life; disconnected from what is sacred; unaware of core values	Preachy/proselytizing; fanatical; rigid values; holier than thou	Connecting with the sacred; pursuing life meaning; finding purpose; expressing virtues

presentations, offering a complement to diagnostic formulation (Hall-Simmonds & McGrath, 2019).

The first empirical study of this model of overuse, underuse, and optimal-use was conducted with clients with and without social anxiety disorder (Freidlin et al., 2017). It found that a particular combination of strength overuses and underuses correctly sorted whether people had social anxiety disorder or not (at an accuracy rate of 87.3%). The combination of overuses/underuses was the overuse of social intelligence and humility, and the underuse of humor, social intelligence (again), self-regulation, and zest. This shows that it *could* be that people with this disorder might be overthinking and over-analyzing the situation (overuse of social intelligence) while over-exerting an attention on others (overuse of humility). At the same time, they might be misreading and miscalculating social cues and nuances (underuse of social intelligence) and bringing too little of a sense of lightheartedness and playfulness (underuse of humor), too little personal passion/energy (underuse of zest), and not engage in balanced self-management (underuse of self-regulation). A second study using this model focused on obsessive-compulsive disorder (Littman-Ovadia & Freidlin, 2019). With this very different disorder, it found a very different pattern of strength overuses and underuses. It found the combination of judgment, social intelligence, appreciation of beauty, fairness, and prudence overused along with the underuse of forgiveness and self-regulation to correctly sort 89.3% of people who have clinical levels of OCD or not. A third study of psychopathology was conducted on borderline personality disorder by Nikki Seligman (2023). Taking a different approach than the previous two, she found that strengths overuse and underuse predicted borderline personality symptoms, noting the underuse of kindness, honesty, self-regulation, prudence, perspective, and love and the overuse of social intelligence, judgment, bravery, curiosity, and zest were independently connected with increased symptoms. Drilling down further, she found a unique profile of overuse/underuse predicted borderline symptoms, namely, the overuse of curiosity along with and underuse of kindness and honesty. Each of these three studies provide empirical support for the overuse, underuse, optimal-use model of Niemiec (2014, 2019). These studies point to what might be *clusters of imbalance* for these well-studied, established disorders. These results need to be replicated before further conclusions are drawn about these disorders or treatment protocols developed, yet point to unique pathways to advance, complement, and support existing research and practice in diagnosing and treating psychopathology.

In addition to these findings, all three empirical studies found that the optimal use of character strengths was significantly associated with flourishing. Character strengths overuse and underuse were independently associated with greater depression and decreased life satisfaction; in addition, the underuse of character strengths was substantially more negatively impacting than the overuse of strengths (Freidlin et al., 2017; Littman-Ovadia & Freidlin, 2019).

The optimal use of character strengths assumes that in each situation of any context, there is a strengths zone or "sweet spot," which can be pursued by counselors and clients for benefits relating to well-being and problem management.

While research on clinical populations is revealing interesting findings and positive benefits (e.g., optimal strengths use), it is likely there are benefits of this reframing for practitioners as well. For example:

- Avoiding stigmatizing individuals with pathology and deficiency.
- Providing an understanding of the individual's resources that can inform treatment planning.
- Suggesting alternate treatments that focus on increasing positive states, not only eliminating negative states.
- Changing treatment from remediation to nurturance of well-being and the resilience effect.
- Encouraging the buffering effect of character strengths.
- Offering more user-friendly language for clients to relate to and that can be made immediately practical (Hall-Simmonds & McGrath, 2019; Niemiec, 2019; Rashid, 2015)

Positive Psychotherapy

Positive psychotherapy (Rashid, 2015) has evolved as one of the more comprehensive ways to introduce character strengths within a psychotherapeutic framework. It uses a variety of interventions to help individuals cultivate positive emotions, thoughts, and behaviors. Some common interventions used in positive psychotherapy include:

1. *Strengths identification*: This involves helping individuals identify and understand their unique character strengths and how they can be used to improve their well-being and relationships with others.
2. *Positive reframing*: This involves helping individuals to reframe negative thoughts and experiences in a more positive light, so they can see their challenges as opportunities for growth.
3. *Gratitude practices*: This involves teaching individuals to cultivate gratitude by focusing on the positive aspects of their lives and expressing appreciation for their blessings.
4. *Mindfulness meditation*: This involves teaching individuals to be present in the moment and cultivate a non-judgmental attitude toward their thoughts and experiences.
5. *Positive relationships*: This involves helping individuals develop and maintain positive relationships with others, so they can experience greater well-being and fulfillment in their lives.
6. *Meaning and purpose*: This involves helping individuals to identify and engage in activities that bring them joy, fulfillment, and a sense of purpose, such as volunteering or pursuing a hobby.
7. *Savoring and positive memories*: This involves helping individuals to focus on and savor positive experiences, so they can build resilience and increase positive emotions.

These interventions are designed to help individuals cultivate positive emotions, thoughts, and behaviors, and increase their overall well-being and sense of fulfillment in life. Tayyab Rashid has observed that well over 50% of positive psychotherapy revolves around character strengths use and practice (Rashid, personal communication, 2011). With positive psychotherapy, a flexible and adaptable approach by the clinician concerning the use of interventions can be tailored to the unique needs and goals of each individual (Rashid & Seligman, 2018).

Positive psychotherapy has been researched in the context of various psychopathologies, and the outcomes have been positive (Slade et al., 2016). It has been shown to be effective in reducing symptoms of depression. Research has shown that incorporating positive interventions, such as gratitude journaling or mindfulness meditation, can help individuals to reframe negative thoughts and cultivate positive emotions, leading to a reduction in symptoms of depression.

1. *Anxiety*: Positive psychotherapy has been shown to be effective in reducing symptoms of anxiety. By focusing on character strengths and positive experiences, individuals can increase their resilience and feel more empowered in the face of life's challenges, leading to a reduction in anxiety symptoms.
2. *Substance abuse*: Positive psychotherapy has been used as a complementary treatment for individuals with substance abuse issues. By promoting positive experiences and character strengths, individuals can develop a stronger sense of purpose and find more meaningful ways to cope with stress, reducing the likelihood of substance abuse.
3. *Post-traumatic stress disorder (PTSD)*: Positive psychotherapy has been shown to be effective in reducing symptoms of PTSD, particularly when used in conjunction with other evidence-based treatments. By helping individuals to identify and develop their character strengths, positive psychotherapy can increase their resilience and ability to cope with trauma-related symptoms.
4. *Psychosis*: Research has shown that recovery from psychosis is also possible using positivepsychotherapy (Slade et al., 2016; Chu et al., 2022).

The Practice

More than cultivating a series of new interventions, a radical shift in perception of the individual treatment approach and measurement are needed to shift the paradigm from deficit to strength-based awareness and intervention. Character strength development is already beginning to shift this paradigm. The emphasis has been on what's wrong rather than on what's strong. By including character strengths in the assessment and treatment plans for psychiatric disabilities, it awakens the practitioner to one of the more sophisticated and widely used tools for improving and maintaining well-being. Using a character strength approach can facilitate relapse prevention while reducing distress, increase development of coping strategies, and provide means and measures for greater balance toward emotional well-being.

Thus, a character strengths approach can be woven into any (and all) elements of psychiatric care. Below are four overarching areas character strengths development can be integrated into traditional psychiatric approaches—initial interview content; development of treatment plans; emphasis on relapse prevention; and increasing subjective well-being.

1. *Intake interviews*. What we notice and ask for in an intake interview determines the trajectory of the treatment. Intake with prospective patients is typically tailored toward problems only, with only a scant exploration of the individual's resources—overlooking potential areas of well-being that exist and are underused. The lack of capitalization on existing strengths and abilities has been missing in favor of diagnosing the problem. This results in a lack of capitalization upon inherent abilities that could be helpful at each stage of treatment. To adequately assess uniform and globally valid strengths is needed to complete the other end of the spectrum. This is what the VIA Survey offers. The *DSM* in its various incarnations has provided a somewhat agreed upon categorization of ailments. The VIA Classification of 24 character strengths provides what Peterson and Seligman (2004) referred to, tongue-in-cheek, as the anti-DSM; for sure, it offers a consensual nomenclature, or common language for positive strengths. The VIA Survey provides a way to identify and assess these universal qualities of well-being. Using the VIA Survey during the initial interview better orients the perception of the treatment provider and the individual in treatment. In this way, the VIA Survey itself becomes a type of intervention in that it shifts or complements what will be attended to during treatment.
2. *Treatment plans*. When deficit identification is the primary (and in most case only) perception of the treatment provider, it skews what is seen and what is excluded from a treatment plan. When we look for deficits in thinking, behavior, and emotions we find them, and their amelioration becomes the goal. What we do not see is the good in someone because we are not looking for or trained to do so. This is a myopic way of approaching the situation. Correction by only treating a malady is ill-fated. To illustrate, 80% of people with depression relapse (Burcusa & Iacono, 2007). This high rate of relapse is reflective of most mental health treatments that take this approach of treating only what is wrong. People get well only to need more assistance. Looking at symptom reduction as the sole measure of wellness will fail to catch features that might hold greater promise for recovery and habilitation. We miss the forest for the trees. In doing so we lose sight of the whole person and the abilities they bring to the situation. Focusing only on what is wrong is an approach that no longer serves humanity. A character strength assessment broadens the lens of targeted features, which can provide elements for upregulation (Niemiec, 2019) and offers a treatment plan that is more comprehensive and life-affirming for the individual. The intake is the foundation for the treatment plan which should include the downregulation of the negative and upregulation of the positive.
3. *Relapse prevention assessment*. Much of the current treatment research emphasizes the treatment effectiveness in reducing the targeted problem. While this

addresses "effectiveness" in one way, it ignores the more important statistic—relapse. Studies focusing on coping with negative emotions and experiences report best results immediately follow treatment. There is a severe drop-off when compared to relapse. As an example, studies show that CBT therapy is also effective for many during the treatment phase, but once the treatment stops, more than half will relapse within the year following, and four out of five of those who do relapse will have that happen within the first 6 months (Ali et al., 2017). The longer past the treatment phase the greater the risk of the changes not being maintained. What worked immediately after treatment begins to wane as time passes and the measure of sustainable treatment interventions takes a backseat to immediate treatment effectiveness for reducing symptoms. Good treatments do not as a rule yield a good long-term result. Character strengths on the other hand have been shown to help stabilize recovery and habilitation efforts. By investing in character strengths development, individuals with psychiatric disabilities are less likely to have their psychiatric symptoms reappear. This means the measure of an effective intervention is not in the treatment, but rather in the way the treatment leads to sustainable changes in emotional self-regulation. Removal of deficits does not make people whole. It makes them less deficient, and typically for only a short time. Improving well-being involves having a framework for acknowledging elements of well-being, using interventions that nurture their emergence, and empowering people to invest their efforts into increasing features that bring more positivity into their life. The VIA Survey assesses and develops character strengths that allow individuals to move toward wholeness and integration rather than only moving away from symptoms. This is what will make their changes endure.

4. *Measures of subjective well-being*. Salutogenesis suggests that the way individuals view their life has an impact, positively or negatively on their health. Following this perspective, the natural outcome of using character strengths from various outcome studies is greater well-being (Schutte & Malouff, 2019). The implication is that a treatment that includes character strengths development will have a positive influence on mental health and well-being because it introduces a positive, proactive stance. Qualitative and quantitative measures that focus on how the use of character strengths aid in the practice of emotional regulation will compliment measures that highlight how suffering has been alleviated.

In the study mentioned in the previous section on the dual role of character strengths for promoting mental health and reducing mental suffering, there were a range of qualitative responses for how each of the 24 character strengths support an individual for mental health during an adversity. A few examples of participant's verbatim responses are borrowed from the study by Niemiec (2023), exhibiting practical ways to turn to character strengths at times of mental suffering:

- *Judgment/critical thinking*: "When faced with difficulties, thinking critically about how to solve problems helps me avoid getting depressed."
- *Kindness*: "Doing for others gives back to me, sometimes in small ways but keeps the focus outward instead of inward thinking my life is so bad."

- *Humility*: "For my mental well-being, I find that uplifting others is as vitally important as seeing them shine and that brings me joy."
- *Appreciation of beauty*: "If I'm having a bad day or am stressed out, looking at something beautiful or unique can snap me out of my mood very quickly."
- *Spirituality*: "Thinking about my purpose and the meaning of everything happens to help me cope with mental illness. It makes me happy to know that all my actions have meaning, and it allows me to move on from hard situations."

Practically speaking, we cannot know what is wrong with a person until we understand what is right. To illustrate this idea, consider a podiatrist treating a patient with a severe limp. The initial evaluation might check all potential causes for the malady, and then the diagnosis would involve determining what was working well as a way of narrowing what is not. When there is a problem, the correction must assess what is subpar, missing, or excessive causing the condition.

But what if the podiatrist saw the limp and decided (without determining what was working well first) that taking the limp away was the proper intervention. She might suggest a cortisol injection, a prescriptive insert, or a pair of orthopedic shoes. These measures might, indeed, bring on relief. But what if eventually these approaches failed? After the injection wore off, or the insert and orthopedic footwear proved unsuccessful, the patient returns with the same limp and says the pain remains. A capricious podiatrist would continue guessing. Perhaps a stronger injection and more elaborate prosthetics would be used. Only if the podiatrist was lucky would this approach to treatment work. This metaphorically is what is happening when we view a psychiatric disability as only a deficiency—an emotional limp if you will. If the treatment applied is aimed at only at correcting what is wrong, we miss the real cause, and as a result use treatments that look like they are effective in the short run, but lead to relapse downstream.

The astute podiatrist looks at what is working well as a way of selecting, then fine-tuning, the treatment. What is not operating optimally would be highlighted while those elements working well would be relied on to continue. This results in finding treatment(s) that do not upset the well-working features. Doing so would not only relieve the pain, but provide a course of action for a sustainable correction.

Consider for a moment where the limping patient's problem might be. It could be an issue with a joint in the ankle or knee, muscle weakness, a blister, tumor, wart, or bunion. It might even be emanating from something amiss in the spine or the result of an injury—perhaps even a fractured bone. If any one of these might be the cause, the injection, insert, or corrective shoes would not provide more than temporary relief. The treatment would seem to work, yet ultimately fail.

We are in a similar position when it comes to the imperfect diagnosability from symptoms with only the *DSM*. If the emotional limp is a cognitive distortion, we do not know if it was caused by a traumatic event that led to PTSD. From a phobia? OCD? Perhaps anxiety and depression are causing it? Or is it a symptom of schizophrenia? Treating the distortion alone does not mean we have made a correction that will last.

But what if the podiatrist offers a thorough intake evaluation asking various questions about the history of the limp? What if exams, X-rays, and tests showed these potential causes were deemed working well, functioning optimally? What might the good podiatrist do then? She might look for other possibilities. What if she discovered that our patient was an avid runner, logging in 20 miles a week for the past several years? How might the diagnosis proceed? Perhaps the foot is being overused. What conditions might ensue from this? Plantar fasciitis and a heel spur might be two conditions aggravated by the constant strain of running. The first, inflammation of the plantar fascia, the band of ligament that runs under the foot from the heel to the toes, could then be evaluated. If that checks out, the heel spur, calcium deposits on the heel bone, could be zeroed in on.

For this metaphor let us say a calcium deposit on the heel is the culprit. Rather than something lacking or deficient, like muscle weakness or a bone fracture, the problem is coming from excess/overuse—not a deficiency/underuse. Too much of something can create conditions that cause pathology. In this instance correcting the overuse while alleviating the pain until this can happen becomes the treatment plan. This can be true with psychiatric disabilities as well.

These provide the foundational framework for understanding psychopathology through the specifics of eunoia. By knowing which character strengths are functioning well, and recognizing traits that indicate an overuse, underuse, or opposite, we get a clearer picture of how to treat the emotional limp.

Consider the concept of the golden mean—the "just right" balance of optimal strengths use. Like a violin string that can be too taut or loose, character strengths can be just right, or out of tune. Mental health and psychological well-being in this theory is generated from the optimal use of character strengths. This can mean that when something is wrong it is because one or more of the 24 character strengths is not operating in the suitable range. Might psychological disorders be explained by clusters of overuse and underuse? Might new explanations of the development of certain conditions be, in part, because of patterns of strengths imbalance?

These ways of looking at imbalance are descriptive—offering hypothetical descriptions that point toward explanations of problems, disorders, and life challenges. There is substantial potential for prescriptive as well. For example, when someone displays a particular trait (such as indifference), ideas for the treatment program become apparent. They need to develop their capacity for kindness.

There are several practical interventions that have been detailed and are theorized to help foster optimal-use and/or manage character strengths overuse and underuse, including direct questioning, reflecting, strengths-spotting, mindfulness, implementation of the Aware-Explore-Apply model, feedback from others, the towing effect, and the tempering effect (Niemiec, 2019). We focus on the latter two next.

Towing effect: The towing effect refers to the boosting up of a character strength with a higher strength one is more accustomed to using. Consider a client wanting to boost up one of their lower strengths that they are underusing; the towing effect occurs when they deliberately turn to one of their most energizing signature strengths to give it that boost (Niemiec, 2019). For example, a client might use their signature strength of curiosity to self-explore new ways they might use more of their lower strength of prudence in their life. Another client might use their signature strength of perspective to tow along their lower strength of bravery by observing courageous people in their life, in the media, and in books and movies. They consider the ways bravery is being used and the advice that any brave person might give them to become more courageous. A practitioner might ask their clients certain questions to support the eliciting of the towing effect:

- How might you take action with one of your top 5 signature strengths to boost one of your lower strengths?
- Think of a situation in which you successfully brought forth one of your typically underused strengths. Which character strength was most involved in giving it a boost?

Tempering effect: The tempering effect refers to the use of a character strength to temper or manage an overused strength. For example, consider a person who is overusing their creativity at a meeting by coming up with so many ideas that it is overwhelming the group. They might turn to their strength of self-regulation to temper their impulse to share the next idea that pops in their head. A person who is overusing their judgment/critical thinking strength by engaging in heavy self-criticism and negative self-talk might temper this strength with forgiveness which is a strength involving letting go and softening intensities. A practitioner might facilitate the tempering effect with a couple of questions:

- Which of your character strengths might help you bring balance to an overused strength? What can you do to take action?
- Think of a situation in which you overused a strength and thus it had a negative impact on someone or yourself. Which character strength might you have used to bring balance or temper that strength overuse? What would that tempering look like?

Case Study

In the Netherlands there is a treatment facility known as Hoeve Boschoord. One of the authors (DT) had the opportunity to work with the staff of the facility in developing treatment programs. This unique facility is a prison, hospital, psychiatric treatment center, farm, and bicycle repair factory. It has a novel approach to the treatment of individuals who have multiple diagnoses. Most of the men incarcerated there have an intellectual disability, a psychiatric disability, and a conduct disorder usually involving a sexual offense.

The closest style of therapy this approach could be likened to is milieu therapy or a therapeutic community. But it is more than that. Hoeve Boschoord typically accepts individuals who have an array of diagnoses with the accompanying symptoms and who need to serve jail time. A typical inmate is placed there due to a sexual and/or drug offense. In the instances the author was involved, the men incarcerated were serving 7-year sentences for their sexual misconduct.

One of the very interesting and unique features of this program is that as people entered the facility to begin serving their sentence, they were very quickly assigned a pigeon or rabbit to take care of. In one of the most rapid therapeutic shifts one could witness, highly volatile, disruptive, violent, and dangerous individuals showed a tremendous affiliation, care, and concern for these small, helpless animals. How did this transformation come about? Three important components provide an answer.

The first is in understanding why being kind to small animals would be considered part of the treatment plan. The inmates in question were both cruel and indifferent by legal standards. They had violated another person's physical well-being and rights without care, and, by definition, they were cruel and indifferent. The display of these symptoms was indicative of a substantial underuse of kindness in many situations. Their behavior indicated they did not have an element of kindness in their life. What these men needed in their life was to be more kind. The correction came from cultivating a strength that was grossly underused.

Secondly, the assignment of a pigeon or a rabbit as they enter the facility might seem like an ill-conceived plan considering their history. However, the well-being of these small animals was tethered to their jail time. If the animal were to die anywhere during the first year of their imprisonment their sentence time would be set back to zero. The men were profoundly motivated to care for the well-being of another life. In other words, the inmate's well-being was directly tied to the care and well-being of another life. Thus, the character strengths of love and appreciation of beauty were directly fostered.

Finally, this was only the first of several interventions that unfolded through their time at Hoeve Boschoord. Each year they were assigned to animals to care for, duties on the farm, even engaging in the assistance of the birth of a calf as part of their therapeutic journey. At each stage the level of their engagement was connected to their own well-being. By caring for others they are caring for themselves. They are tapping into character strengths of humanity and justice, as well as temperance and transcendence. This was supported by a heavy emphasis on group therapy as well as the milieu component emphasizing they were part of a larger community that was there to support them as they needed to become aware of their need to support the community.

Curiously, this unique program with an emphasis on cultivating the "better angels of our nature" has been shown to be as one of the most effective programs in the treatment of recidivism.

Future Directions

While we have highlighted a range of important concepts and interesting research findings, there is far more unknown about the interplay of character strengths and mental affliction or psychopathology than known. As models and frameworks are revised or developed, there is a substantial need for clinical studies in these areas. Randomized intervention studies of single character strengths interventions would help to build the armamentarium of practitioners helping clients. Such studies would feed future multi-step programs involving character strengths for particular populations in need, such as programs for depression or anxiety.

One area ripe with potential is the understanding of each psychological disorder through the lens of strengths overuse and underuse patterns. As disorders become more clearly understood—and partially or fully explained—by these phenomena, new opportunities emerge. Replication of that research is needed and treatment protocols that utilize the tempering and towing effects could follow. Such programs might not be a replacement for other treatments, rather would provide a comparable alternative or an adjunct to existing treatments.

Key Takeaways

- The history of psychology's treatment of psychiatric disabilities has largely focused on alleviating suffering.
- As mental health issues become problematic largely due to their persistence, a treatment plan should be layered in its approach. Both pain and potentiality need to be part of the assessment with the goal to find ways to have these interventions produce sustainable changes.
- In addition to downregulating negative emotions and symptoms, separate interventions are needed to upregulate positive emotions with the goal tipping the scale in favor of thriving and flourishing.
- The character strength approach is a salutogenetic framework.
- Numerous studies have found character strengths provide a substantial and important buffering effect for mental illnesses and for mental vulnerabilities.
- Research has found that the character strengths perceived as most important for creating good mental health are love, kindness, curiosity, creativity, and perspective.
- Research has found that individuals prefer to use their character strengths for emotional coping at difficult times, as opposed to using character strengths for behavioral action or changes in thinking.
- Treatments and measurement are needed to shift the paradigm from deficit-based to strength-based awareness and intervention. This can happen by changing the nature of intake interviews, treatment plans, relapse prevention goals, and including measures of well-being.
- Character strengths can be viewed as being overused, underused, and optimally used in any situation within any context.
- Optimal-use of character strengths has been positively correlated to life satisfaction and flourishing, and negatively correlated to depression. Likewise, suboptimal (underuse and overuse) are significantly related to higher depression and less flourishing and life satisfaction. Initial patterns for social anxiety disorder, obsessive-compulsive disorder, and borderline personality disorder have been found by researchers.

- Positive psychotherapy is a comprehensive therapeutic approach to introduce and work with character strengths and other positive phenomena.
- The towing effect of character strengths refers to the use of a signature strength to boost another strength (usually an "underused" strength). The tempering effect refers to the use of one character strength to balance or temper an overused strength.

References

Ali, S., Rhodes, L., Moreea, O., McMillan, D., Gilbody, S., Leach, C., et al. (2017). How durable is the effect of low-intensity C.B.T. for depression and anxiety? Remission and relapse in a longitudinal cohort study. *Behaviour Research and Therapy, 94*, 1–8.

Antonovsky, A. (1979). *Health, stress, and coping. New perspectives on mental and physical well-being* (pp. 12–37). Jossey-Bass.

Aristotle. (2000). *Nicomachean ethics* (R. Crisp, Trans.). Cambridge University Press (Original work composed 4th century BCE).

Burcusa, S. L., & Iacono, W. G. (2007). Risk for recurrence in depression. *Clinical Psychology Review, 27*(8), 959–985.

Cheng, X., Bu, H., Duan, W., He, A., & Zhang, Y. (2020). Measuring character strengths as possible protective factors against suicidal ideation in older Chinese adults: A cross-sectional study. *BMC Public Health, 20*. https://doi.org/10.1186/s12889-020-8457-7

Chiesa, A., Serretti, A., & Jakobsen, J. C. (2013). Mindfulness: Top–down or bottom–up emotion regulation strategy? *Clinical Psychology Review, 33*(1), 82–96. http://www.azmonyar.com/DownloadPDF/57782853.pdf

Chu, M. H. W., Lau, B., Leung, J., Chan, S. C., Tang, B., Lau, C., et al. (2022). Positive psychotherapy for psychosis in Hong Kong: A randomized controlled trial. *Schizophrenia Research, 240*, 175–183.

Datu, J., & Niemiec, R. M. (2023). *Disability: Character strengths, stigma, and acceptance across different disabilities*. Data from 21,800 people, collected on the VIA Institute on Character website.

De Witte, N. A., Sütterlin, S., Braet, C., & Mueller, S. C. (2017). Psychophysiological correlates of emotion regulation training in adolescent anxiety: Evidence from the novel PIER task. *Journal of Affective Disorders, 214*, 89–96. https://biblio.ugent.be/publication/8526865

Demirci, İ., Ekşi, H., Ekşi, F., & Kaya, C. (2019). Character strengths and psychological vulnerability: The mediating role of resilience. *Current Psychology*. https://doi.org/10.1007/s12144-019-00533-1

Eippert, F., Veit, R., Weiskopf, N., Erb, M., Birbaumer, N., & Anders, S. (2007). Regulation of emotional responses elicited by threat-related stimuli. *Human Brain Mapping, 28*(5), 409–423. https://onlinelibrary.wiley.com/doi/full/10.1002/hbm.20291

Fredrickson, B. L. (2004). Gratitude, like other positive emotions, broadens and builds. *The Psychology of Gratitude, 145*, 166.

Freidlin, P., Littman-Ovadia, H., & Niemiec, R. M. (2017). Positive psychopathology: Social anxiety via character strengths underuse and overuse. *Personality and Individual Differences, 108*, 50–54.

Hall-Simmonds, A., & McGrath, R. E. (2019). Character strengths and clinical presentation. *The Journal of Positive Psychology, 14*(1), 51–60.

Huta, V., & Hawley, L. (2010). Psychological strengths and cognitive vulnerabilities: Are they two ends of the same continuum or do they have independent relationships with well-being and ill-being? *Journal of Happiness Studies, 11*, 71–93.

Iwamoto, S. K., Alexander, M., Torres, M., Irwin, M. R., Christakis, N. A., & Nishi, A. (2020). Mindfulness meditation activates altruism. *Scientific reports, 10*(1), 6511.

Katsumi, Y., & Dolcos, S. (2020). Suppress to feel and remember less: Neural correlates of explicit and implicit emotional suppression on perception and memory. *Neuropsychologia, 145*, 106683.

Littman-Ovadia, H., & Freidlin, P. (2019). Positive psychopathology and positive Functioning: OCD, flourishing and satisfaction with life through the lens of character strength underuse, overuse and optimal use. *Applied Research in Quality of Life*. https://doi.org/10.1007/s11482-018-9701-5

Livingstone, K. M., & Srivastava, S. (2012). Up-regulating positive emotions in everyday life: Strategies, individual differences, and associations with positive emotion and well-being. *Journal of Research in Personality, 46*(5), 504–516.

McTiernan, K., Gullon-Scott, F., & Dudley, R. (2020). An exploration of strength use and its relationship with life satisfaction, positive self-beliefs and paranoid ideation. *International Journal of Wellbeing, 10*(2), 53–70.

Neff, K. D. (2003). Self-compassion: An alternative conceptualization of a healthy attitude toward oneself. *Self and Identity, 2*, 85–101.

Niemiec, R. M. (2014). Mindfulness and character strengths: A practical guide to flourishing. Hogrefe.

Niemiec, R. M. (2019). Finding the golden mean: the overuse, underuse, and optimal use of character strengths. *Counselling Psychology Quarterly, 32*(3–4), 453–471.

Niemiec, R. M. (2020). Six functions of character strengths for thriving at times of adversity and opportunity: A theoretical perspective. *Applied Research in Quality of Life, 15*, 551–572. https://doi.org/10.1007/s11482-018-9692-2

Niemiec, R. M. (2023). Mental health and character strengths: The dual-role of boosting well-being and reducing suffering. *Mental Health and Social Inclusion*. https://doi.org/10.1108/MHSI-01-2023-0012

Ormel, J., Hollon, S. D., Kessler, R. C., Cuijpers, P., & Monroe, S. M. (2022). More treatment but no less depression: The treatment-prevalence paradox. *Clinical Psychology Review, 91*, 102111.

Peterson, C. (2006). The values in action (VIA) classification of strengths. In M. Csikszentmihalyi & L. Csikszentmihalyi (Eds.), *A life worth living: Contributions to positive psychology* (pp. 29–48). Oxford University Press.

Prince, M., Patel, V., Saxena, S., Maj, M., Maselko, J., Phillips, M. R., & Rahman, A. (2007). No health without mental health. *The lancet, 370*(9590), 859–877.

Quoidbach, J., Mikolajczak, M., & Gross, J. J. (2015). Positive interventions: An emotion regulation perspective. *Psychological Bulletin, 141*(3), 655.

Rashid, T. (2015). Positive psychotherapy: A strength-based approach. *The Journal of Positive Psychology, 10*(1), 25–40. https://doi.org/10.1080/17439760.2014.920411

Rashid, T., & Seligman, M. P. (2018). *Positive psychotherapy: Clinician manual*. Oxford University Press.

Rubin-Falcone, H., Weber, J., Kishon, R., Ochsner, K., Delaparte, L., Doré, B., et al. (2018). Longitudinal effects of cognitive behavioral therapy for depression on the neural correlates of emotion regulation. *Psychiatry Research: Neuroimaging, 271*, 82–90.

Salzberg, S. (1995). *Lovingkindness: The revolutionary art of happiness*. Shambhala.

Schutte, N. S., & Malouff, J. M. (2019). The impact of signature character strengths interventions: A meta-analysis. *Journal of Happiness Studies, 20*, 1179–1196.

Seligman, M. E. (2015). Chris Peterson's unfinished masterwork: The real mental illnesses. *The Journal of Positive Psychology, 10*(1), 3–6.

Seligman, N. (2023). *The underuse and overuse of character strengths in borderline personality disorder symptoms*. ETD Collection for Fordham University. AAI28774578. https://research.library.fordham.edu/dissertations/AAI28774578

Seligman, M. E., & Csikszentmihalyi, M. (2000). *Positive psychology: An introduction* (Vol. 55, No. 1, p. 5). American Psychological Association.

Silton, R. L., Kahrilas, I. J., Skymba, H. V., Smith, J., Bryant, F. B., & Heller, W. (2020). Regulating positive emotions: Implications for promoting well-being in individuals with depression. *Emotion, 20*(1), 93.

Slade, M., Brownell, T., Rashid, T., & Schrank, B. (2016). *Positive psychotherapy for psychosis: A clinician's guide and manual*. Routledge.

Sueki, H. (2020). What character strengths are protective factors for suicidal ideation?: A cross-sectional study in Japan. *Psychology, Health & Medicine*. https://doi.org/10.1080/13548506.2020.1758334

Waters, L., Algoe, S. B., Dutton, J., Emmons, R., Fredrickson, B. L., Heaphy, E., Moskowitz, J. T., Neff, K., Niemiec, R. M., Pury, C., & Steger, M. (2021). Positive psychology in a pandemic: Buffering, bolstering, and building mental health. *Journal of Positive Psychology*. https://doi.org/10.1080/17439760.2021.1871945

Zaehringer, J., Jennen-Steinmetz, C., Schmahl, C., Ende, G., & Paret, C. (2020). Psychophysiological effects of downregulating negative emotions: Insights from a meta-analysis of healthy adults. *Frontiers in Psychology, 11*, 470.

Seligman, M. E. P., & Csikszentmihalyi, M. (2000). *Positive psychology: An introduction* (Vol. 55, No. 1, p. 5). American Psychological Association.

[illegible]

[illegible]

[illegible]

[illegible]

[illegible]

Chapter 7
Physical and Medical Disorders and Character Strengths

Strength does not come from physical capacity. It comes from an indomitable will.

-Mahatma Gandhi.

The Concepts

Health is more than the absence of disease (Seligman, 2008). Character strengths have a critical role in both creating health and disease management (Niemiec & Yarova, 2018). A variety of important functions for character strengths have been theorized in regard to both the boosting of well-being opportunities and the managing of adverse situations, such as cultivating resilience (Niemiec, 2019a). These sets of well-being and adversity functions play a clear and important role when an individual is experiencing a physical condition or diagnosable medical disorder.

In *JAMA*, the flagship journal of the medical field, the argument has been made for character as one of the key elements of flourishing for patients and patient care in medical/healthcare settings (VanderWeele, 2019).

Physical disability pertains to illnesses that impair an individual's ability to move and maintain stamina in physical activities, for example, conditions such as congenital bone deformities, arthritis, cerebral palsy, spinal cord injuries, multiple sclerosis. The stigmatization of such conditions that occurs is lessened by exposure to people with physical disabilities. There are high correlations for people high in the character strengths of kindness, fairness, social intelligence, and love of learning (also perspective, appreciation of beauty, and curiosity) and less stigmatization, while self-regulation, perseverance, and spirituality are strongly associated with higher stigmatization (Datu & Niemiec, 2023). Character strengths provide a language of humanness and connection to suffering.

Chronic illness and disability (CID) have long been the central focus of rehabilitation psychology. The alignment and overlap with a positive psychosocial adaptation to disability suggests that character strength development may be a highly relevant and important addition to rehabilitation psychology's toolbox (Livneh & Martz, 2016).

R. M. Niemiec, D. Tomasulo, *Character Strengths and Abilities Within Disabilities*, Positive Psychology and Disability Series,
https://doi.org/10.1007/978-3-031-36294-1_7

The Science

There are a number of studies that have been conducted with physical conditions and medical conditions, although no particular condition or diagnosis has received extensive examination through the character strengths lens. We review several examples looking at different conditions in turn.

Heart disease: A couple of studies by Huffman et al. (2011, 2016) looked at cardiac patients from an intervention perspective. They found that patients suffering from acute coronary syndrome benefitted from an 8-week phone intervention which included identifying and using a signature strength. They also found that the combined use of three character strengths (gratitude, hope, and kindness) brought increases in health-related quality of life compared to a relaxation group and to controls. In a large study of 481 open-heart surgery patients, another set of researchers examined character strengths (hope and spirituality) and a number of daily living activities after surgery. They found that those who pursued pre-surgery positive spiritual/religious coping had better functioning/activities of daily living. They concluded that pre-surgery positive spiritual coping may have played an important role in better functioning/recovery following surgery (Ai et al., 2021).

Lung disease: A large-scale study using epidemiological data examined the character strength of honesty/integrity in nearly 10,000 older adults. It found that after 4-year follow-up, those higher in honesty/integrity had an 18% lower risk of lung disease, 11% lower risk of depression, and less difficulties with mobility and daily living activities (Weziak-Bialowolska et al., 2021).

Fibromyalgia: In a study of over 400 people with fibromyalgia, the researchers highlight a finding that finding silver linings was critical in regard to the connection between illness impairment and depression. They suggest a central strategy for patients as identifying positive qualities such as using signature strengths interventions to support treatment (Hirsch et al., 2019).

Chronic pain: In two studies of character strengths and coping with pain, the character strength most associated with pain self-efficacy was zest. A follow-up study offered a zest intervention involving writing about different ways to use zest each day and found the intervention improved pain self-efficacy as well as the capacity to function despite pain (Graziosi et al., 2020). A small study of chronic back pain patients found that a character strengths and gratitude intervention led to improved daily happiness and less daily anger (Baxter et al., 2012).

Brain injury: A study by Hanks et al. (2014) examined a group of patients with traumatic brain injury and found that character strengths and virtues showed unique value in predicting physical health and disability. Character strengths, resilience, and positive mood were related to primary factors of treatment success (including treatment expectations and perception of functional ability) in rehabilitation medicine settings among a group of individuals with acquired brain injury (Bertisch et al., 2014). In a randomized intervention study of individuals with traumatic brain injuries, the character strengths interventions group was found to be superior to the control group on measures of happiness and mood (Andrewes et al., 2014).

Pediatric illness: In a study of children with a life-threatening illness, it was found that higher benefit-finding and character strengths (i.e., love and gratitude) predicted positive changes in life satisfaction over time. In turn, positive emotions predicted changes in benefit-finding over time through various character strengths such as zest and gratitude (Chaves et al., 2016a, b). Several of these researchers also studied a positive intervention (i.e., granting a wish) among seriously ill children, compared to a waitlist control group, and found the intervention group to have increased levels of strengths, life satisfaction, positive emotions, and less nausea (Chaves et al., 2016a, b).

Multiple sclerosis: Smedema (2020) examined 624 people with multiple sclerosis and found the character strengths that had the strongest association with quality of life (QoL) were zest, hope, and spirituality. Disability was not a mediator for strengths and QoL. The most endorsed character strengths were honesty, kindness, and fairness. The researcher concluded character strengths enhance the QoL of people with multiple sclerosis directly and through an influence on the negative effects of the disease.

Surgical recovery: A case study examined a patient suffering after eye surgery and offered character strengths interventions. The intervention focused on identifying and appreciating strengths, reviewing success stories and peak experiences with strengths, and implementation intentions with strengths (Shinichiro et al., 2018).

General chronic illnesses: There have been several studies of character strengths with chronic illnesses in general, and thereby a rigorous review was conducted. The focus was clinical studies on character strengths-based interventions for patients with chronic illnesses. The results showed these interventions boosted self-esteem and self-efficacy and reduced depression (Yan et al., 2020). Another review of positive interventions in chronic illness patients suggested the strengths of gratitude and kindness as two of the most frequent areas for intervention focus and a need to target other strengths with these populations such as perseverance, love, and hope (Ghosh & Deb, 2017). Other research has found that when an individual has a physical disorder, there is less of a toll on life satisfaction if they are high on the character strengths of bravery, kindness, and humor (Peterson et al., 2006). Other well-being connections have been found with a range of specific character strengths, such as the strength of gratitude being linked with higher well-being among those with neuromuscular disease (Emmons & McCullough, 2003).

COVID-19: A group of positive psychology leaders got together to offer the best practical strategies to better handle adversity during the pandemic. They focused on a range of well-being topics (including character strengths) for the purpose of buffering mental illness and bolstering mental health (Waters et al., 2021). Articles have offered practical strategies for using character strengths to boost coping and reappraise challenges particularly during COVID-19 (Rashid & McGrath, 2020).

A number of empirical studies in various countries have been conducted during the pandemic of COVID-19 and examining character strengths as a critical factor in well-being. A large international study examined individuals before and during COVID-19 and found a small increase in 17 character strengths. It also found that social support brought a small increase in many character strengths—love, prudence, curiosity, forgiveness, gratitude, honesty, hope, judgment, leadership, humility, and zest (Amoury-Naddaf & Lavy, 2022). In a controlled study of Filipino students during the adversity of the COVID-19 pandemic, students experiencing character strengths interventions (i.e., kindness or gratitude) had significantly higher positive emotions than those in the control group (Datu et al., 2021). An Italian study during COVID-19 in 2020 found that character strengths (as a whole) had a significant direct effect on both mental health and post-traumatic growth; in addition the virtue of transcendence was uniquely related to mental health while the virtue of humanity was uniquely related to post-traumatic growth (Casali et al., 2021). A second Italian study during the COVID-19 pandemic lockdown found the character strengths of hope, zest, prudence, love, and forgiveness were most negatively associated with distress while appreciation of beauty/excellence was significantly positively related to distress. In addition, love and zest were most connected to self-efficacy; and zest with general mental health (Casali et al., 2020). A Greek study during COVID-19 found that the character strengths of love, curiosity, perseverance, hope, and zest were associated with well-being during quarantine (Vasileiou et al., 2021). In a COVID-19 patient from Spain, all character strengths groupings/factors predicted an increase in mental health and positive emotions (with the exception of strengths of restraint for the latter outcome). Character strengths of restraint, interpersonal, and fortitude predicted a decrease in negative affect (Martinez-Marti et al., 2020).

Another study looked at 269 individuals with chronic health conditions and disabilities experiencing COVID-19 stress. The researchers found multiple character strengths significantly and independently moderated the relationship between COVID-19 stress and well-being (Umucu et al., 2020). In a study of 617 adolescents, character strengths served as a protective factor that moderated the relationship between COVID-19 stress and depression symptoms (Liu & Wang, 2021).

General physical disabilities: One study looked at 51 participants in China with a variety of (largely acquired) physical disabilities exposed to awareness and use of their strengths. When compared to 22 individuals in a control group, those able to use their strengths improved their level of flourishing as they were coping with living with their disability. In a 3-month follow-up it was determined that when compared to the control group those exposed to the character-strength well-being intervention showed greater resilience. Importantly, the initial effects of the strength-based approach were not significant—but the postintervention period was. This suggests that the intervention may have a type of sleeper-effect, promoting continuation of a positive adaptation by cultivating resilience (Bu & Duan, 2021).

The Practice

There are a number of studies showing the importance of "creating health" and linking character strengths with healthy lifestyle and health behaviors. This can be distinct from or in tandem with approaches focused on reducing symptoms or disease. In this section, we discuss practices for both creating health and managing disease as well as interventions that can target medical and healthcare professionals.

Increasing Health

We begin by highlighting some of the pioneering research on the connection between character strengths and health. The largest study on this topic involved 60,000 subjects from 159 countries and found numerous links between character strengths and health-related quality of life, purpose, and health behaviors, including Niemiec's (2019b) five pillars of health—healthy eating, sleep, activity/exercise, socializing, and self-care. Across health-related quality of life outcomes, the strengths of zest, self-regulation, hope, and gratitude were the strongest associations, with zest and self-regulation as strongest across health behaviors (Weziak-Bialowolska et al., 2023).

When approximately 9000 people were asked to select one of the 24 character strengths they have found to be most important when they are physically unwell, the highest strength reported was perseverance (11% of participants). The strengths of hope, love, self-regulation, and humor rounded out the top 5 (Niemiec, 2023). This points to five immediate internal resources—or personal interventions—an individual might turn to in order to cope with or overcome physical struggles. There is the energy of overcoming the many physical and mental obstacles and bodily ails (perseverance), the discipline to focus on caring for the body (self-regulation and love), the playfulness and laughter about one's situation and being not fully in control (humor), and the optimism to look positively to the future despite suffering in the present (hope).

Other studies have linked character strengths with a myriad of health behaviors such as having an active way of life, healthy eating, watching one's food intake, and physical fitness. All character strengths (except humility and spirituality) were associated with multiple health behaviors. While self-regulation had the highest associations overall, curiosity, appreciation of beauty/excellence, gratitude, hope, and humor also displayed strong connections with health behaviors (Proyer et al., 2013). Physical health has also been shown to be crucially linked in large-scale studies in developing (i.e., majority world) nations. For example, in randomized controlled trials involving thousands of girls in poverty in India, girls who received a curriculum which incorporated character strengths (identification and use of signature strengths and concrete examples of other strengths) exhibited significantly greater physical health (and psychosocial health) benefits in comparison to those girls who received a similar curriculum which did not include character strengths as well as a control group (Leventhal et al., 2015, 2016). In addition, across eating, exercising, and working, a set of almost all character strengths were beneficially related to competence, relatedness, and autonomy (Stuntz, 2018).

In a 2023 study, routine exercise as well as higher levels were able to predict greater resilience following a stressor. It was also found that consistent moderate levels of exercise improved depression scores. For those whose depression increased or remained high there was reduced exercise following a stressor. Exercise may both buffer depression and promote resilience (Szuhany et al., 2023).

With these studies as a foundation, there are a myriad of practical strategies for connecting character strengths and health. We turn to the five pillars of health model (Niemiec, 2019b), and the descriptions and findings from Weziak-Bialowolska et al. (2021), as shown in Table 7.1. In some cases, the descriptions (in the study and in the table) are more narrow than what the breadth and depth of the pillar offers (e.g.,

Table 7.1 The 5 pillars of health and highest character strength associations

5 Pillars of health	Description	Top 5 character strength connections
Healthy eating/drinking	Generally viewed as eating a diet with a lot of fruits and vegetables and foods with plenty of essential nutrients; managing the intake of unhealthy foods (such as sweets, trans fats, high calorie drinks, and eating at fast-food restaurants); managing the quantity of food/drink each day (not too much, not too little); and drinking plenty of water.	Self-regulation, curiosity, appreciation of beauty, hope, honesty
Healthy exercise/activity	Engaging in moderate to vigorous aerobic activities for 150 min per week; and/or at least 2 days of muscle strengthening activities with various muscle groups.	Zest, self-regulation, leadership, perseverance, curiosity
Healthy sleep	Getting sufficient rest each night.	Zest, hope, self-regulation forgiveness, prudence
Healthy socializing	Generally viewed as having daily social connections with family, friends, and/or neighbors/community that is meaningful and mutually beneficial (there is a positive give and take in the conversation or activity). It involves having fun, connecting with others, and feeling some sense of belonging.	Zest, curiosity, hope, love, teamwork
Healthy self-care	Generally viewed as engaging in regular practices or activities that help you feel refreshed, focused, calm/peaceful, connected, more aware, or more in control of stress/tension. Some examples include mindfulness, actively using your character strengths, engaging with your hobbies/interests, walking in nature, relaxation strategies, mind-body strategies, yoga, giving yourself quiet time, journaling, peaceful reflection, prayer, spiritual rituals, and/or loving-kindness practice.	Hope, zest, self-regulation, perspective

the pillars for sleep and exercise); this was done for scientific clarity and measurement purposes in the study.

Based on Table 7.1, we suggest several character strengths interventions. In most of the areas, zest, self-regulation, and hope are facilitative components. We discuss research and interventions to facilitate each.

Zest

Recent research has suggested that regular exercise may be a good way to help ameliorate the impact of depression as well as cope with major life stressors. Stressful events, ongoing coping, and systematic depletion of energy can be challenged and even corrected by using exercise as a direct way to facilitate zest (Szuhany et al., 2023). Other research suggests that as little as 20 min of activity is enough to reap the benefits of exercise (Reycraft et al., 2020). While it is beyond the scope of this chapter to explore all the avenues through which exercise can be achieved, suggestions on how to cultivate exercise habits are ubiquitous. The Mayo Clinic are offered useful examples (Mayo Foundation for Medical Education and Research, 2022a, 2022b).

Cultivation of healthy sleep patterns is one of the best ways to restore, replenish, and refresh your energy. Sleep hygiene typically involves establishing a regular routine and time to retire. Eating no sooner than a few hours before sleeping, not working while in bed, and not consuming caffeine later in the evening can facilitate good sleep. Insufficient sleep can cause a higher expenditure of energy, greater calorie intake, and obesity—all of which deplete zest (Chaput et al., 2023).

Self-Regulation

The key to self-regulation is cultivating ways to facilitate mechanisms that support deliberate and explicit controls that lead to implicit regulation. Research using neuroimaging techniques demonstrate that meditation improves activation and connectivity in areas of the brain related to self-regulation. Regular meditation appears to improve self-regulation over the lifespan (Tang et al., 2014).

Two of the popular, evidence-based, mindfulness meditation programs that cultivate self-regulation are mindfulness-based stress reduction (MBSR) and mindfulness-based strengths practice (MBSP). In one study, 276 adults were compared using the 8-week MBSR program to patients who took escitalopram, the generic name of the anti-anxiety drug Lexapro. The researchers found both interventions worked equally well in reducing severe anxiety symptoms by about 20% (Hoge et al., 2023). MBSP is also an 8-week program. It integrates mindfulness and character strengths and is showing good research outcomes (Bretherton & Niemiec, 2019; Whelan-Berry & Niemiec, 2021), with applications for ethical and personal development (Baer, 2015; Niemiec, 2012), workplace/organizations (Pang & Ruch, 2019), schools/education (Lottman et al., 2017; Wingert et al., 2020), and disability populations (Shogren et al., 2017). The appeal of this method is the mutual synergy of mindfulness/mindful living and character strengths, as well as the benefits showing superiority of MBSP over MBSR for well-being and other outcomes (e.g., Monzani et al., 2021).

Hope

Hope involves goals that we believe we have the ability to achieve (agency) and plans (pathways) on how to attain them (Snyder et al., 1991). Hope interventions centering around the positive experiences of having attained goals through agency and pathways have been successfully used to improve psychological and physical symptoms associated with cancer (Chan et al., 2019). Evidence-based hope therapy exists with the goals of instilling and increasing hope that has strong sustained outcomes (Cheavens & Guter, 2018).

One intervention uses micro-goals to facilitate a sense of hopefulness (Tomasulo, 2020). A micro-goal is an identified small, targeted goal that can be accomplished in a brief period of time. Moving to New York City might be a macro-goal, while taking a half hour to look for one-bedroom apartments for lease is a micro-goal. Hope is bidirectional in that a small bit of positivity about attaining a goal gives you sufficient agency and pathways to attain it. Once achieved, the positive experience is reinforced by the accomplishment. When you use micro-goals, they stimulate the positive experiences of goal-setting, and motivation and means to achieve goals. Other intervention for increasing hopefulness can be found in Tomasulo's work (2020).

Managing Disease

The cultivation of strength-based practices may be one of the greatest ways to facilitate prevention of, and coping with, chronic concerns. As the preceding sample of healthy pillars and their interventions show, finding ways to specifically facilitate strengths in the management of ongoing diseases would not only appear to be helpful strategies in and of themselves, but also accelerants and facilitators of ongoing treatment. A meta-analysis of eight studies involving 692 patients indicated that character strengths-based interventions improved not only the self-esteem and self-efficacy of patients with chronic illnesses, it also reduced their depression (Yan et al., 2020).

A study out of the Human Flourishing Program at Harvard University's Institute for Quantitative Social Science took data from the Health and Retirement Study (HRS). They concluded that hope may be one of the most potent traits to cultivate as we mature. The researchers looked at nearly 13,000 participants with an average age of 66 years. In this study, those with the highest measures of hope in their lives were found to live longer, have fewer chronic conditions, less cancer, lower chronic pain, and less sleep problems. Additionally, they had much higher life satisfaction, sense of purpose in their life, lower psychological stress, more positivity, and better relationships. Those with lower hope had an elevated risk of anxiety, depression, and post-traumatic stress disorder. Having and cultivating hope may be the best emotional prophylactic against a difficult tomorrow (Long et al., 2020).

Supporting Healthcare/Medical Professionals

There are many types of practitioners who work with people with physical disorders and medical conditions. The domain of medicine and the many medical professionals from physicians, nurses, medical assistants, and residents has received some examination from a character strengths lens.

Physicians have been studied in a number of experiments, many from Austria. Studies of hospital physicians have revealed numerous character strengths connections with well-being, in particular hope with thriving, zest with work engagement and less emotional exhaustion, and perseverance and leadership with less depersonalization (Kachel et al., 2021) as well as autonomy (Strecker et al., 2019), and psychological well-being (Huber et al., 2019). While the strengths of humility, social intelligence, and teamwork consistently showed lower correlations, all were reported in interviews as important for well-being at work, especially humility (Kachel et al., 2021). Another study of hospital physicians with 6-month follow-up found a mutual positive impact of signature strengths application and perceived socio-moral climate (Höge et al., 2019). Huber et al. (2020) took the approach of examining the character strengths profiles of various medical professionals. They found medical students and physicians to be highest on the strengths of fairness, honesty, judgment, kindness, and love, and that general surgeons were higher on honesty and prudence and were higher than that of psychiatrists.

Among medical students and resident physicians, the use of signature strengths at work was positively linked with well-being and mental health but not with physical health (Hausler et al. 2017). In Australia, medical students who completed a course that integrated the VIA Classification in a clinical context using personal narratives, experiential exercises, contemplative practices, and reflective practices. The students self-reported improved understanding of the virtues and their importance to the practice of medicine (Seoane et al., 2016). For nurses, the research has focused on rationale, concepts, research review, and interventions that nurses might use to support patients (e.g., Macfarlane, 2019, 2022).

Reducing Burnout

A meta-analysis in 2016 declared physician burnout at epidemic levels (West et al., 2016). More recent research indicates it remains the case (Johns et al., 2022). In response to the need for greater kindness and compassion among healthcare workers, the Compassion Cultivation Training, an 8-week contemplative program, was developed at Stanford University. Using didactic methods, discussions, and evidence-based meditation techniques, the program strives for professional healthcare workers to not only cultivate compassion for others but for themselves (Department of Psychiatry and Behavioral Sciences, n.d.).

Developing the character strength of kindness is more than platitudes about being kind to others, or feeling better about yourself. Based on over 200 studies, the term "compassionomics" has evolved to suggest the kindness conveyed by healthcare workers may be beneficial for the patients, healthcare system, and the healthcare provider alike (Trzeciak et al., 2017). As an example, for patients it has been shown to reduce stress, inflammation, and increase the placebo effect. For healthcare systems there are fewer medical errors, lower costs, and better clinical outcomes. And healthcare providers find better stress buffering and higher self-esteem. As this work continues to evolve, we suggest the inclusion and integration of character strengths approaches, models, and interventions into compassionomics, such as the turning of character strengths both *inwardly* for self-care and self-development and *outwardly* to bring benefit to others (Niemiec, 2018).

Future Directions

The integration of character strengths to examine the causes, correlates, and interventions with distinct medical and physical disabilities is a complex area. In considering areas of future study, we attempt to show the breadth and depth with a range of questions of interest:

- How might character strengths overuse and character strengths underuse cause or contribute to physical disabilities? How might they exacerbate existing conditions?
- What are the character strengths correlates with successful diabetes management? With resilience having a terminal diagnosis?
- Which character strength is best intervened upon to help people cope with heart disease? With a spinal cord injury? What is the role of signature strengths with these and other conditions?
- How might the popular interventions on using signature strengths be applied to improving sleep, coping with post-surgery problems, or overcoming a gastrointestinal problem like irritable bowel syndrome?
- Are signature strengths applications important for fostering each of the 5 pillars of health? With which pillar is the impact most clear?
- Would a randomized study that focuses on the top correlates of one or all of the 5 pillars of health be an effective intervention? If so, for which patients might it best help?
- What is the impact of a physician, nurse, or other medical professional using their signature strengths in their interactions with patients? With their medical team? What impact might that have on the medical culture?

- How might character strengths interventions be brought to a larger scale for wider impact on patients?
- How might character strengths interventions be integrated into compassion-based approaches to engender optimal benefit for clients and healthcare providers?

Key Takeaways

- Health is more than the absence of disease. Character strengths have a critical role in both creating health and disease management.
- Character strength development may be a highly relevant and important addition to rehabilitation psychology's toolbox.
- A wide variety of medical and physical conditions have been researched although no particular condition or diagnosis has received extensive examination through the character strengths lens.
- Five pillars of health have been observed for healthy living, and character strengths form an important foundation: healthy eating, sleep, activity/exercise, socializing, and self-care.
- Across health-related quality of life outcomes, the strengths of zest, self-regulation, hope, and gratitude were the strongest associations, with zest and self-regulation as strongest across health behaviors.
- Exercise and sleep hygiene to cultivate zest, MBSR and MBSP programs to facilitate self-regulation, and micro-goals to foster hope were discussed as character strength interventions.
- Managing disease might be positively impacted by cultivating character strengths; the strength of hope in later years is correlated with living longer, having fewer chronic conditions, less cancer, lower chronic pain, fewer sleep problems, higher life satisfaction, sense of purpose in their life, lower psychological stress, more positivity, and better relationships.
- Among medical students and resident physicians, the use of signature strengths at work was positively linked with well-being and mental health.
- Compassionomics has evolved to suggest the kindness conveyed by healthcare workers may be beneficial for the patients, healthcare system, and the healthcare provider alike.

References

Ai, A. L., Fincham, F. D., & Carretta, H. (2021). ADL and IADL following open-heart surgery: The role of a character strength factor and preoperative medical comorbidities. *Journal of Religion and Health*. https://doi.org/10.1007/s10943-020-01146-w

Amoury-Naddaf, S., & Lavy, S. (2022). Character strengths development in COVID-19 pandemic: Exploring change in turbulent times. *Journal of Happiness Studies, 24*, 185–210.

Andrewes, H. E., Walker, V., & O'Neill, B. (2014). Exploring the use of positive psychology interventions in brain injury survivors with challenging behavior. *Brain Injury, 28*(7), 965–971.

Baer, R. (2015). Ethics, values, virtues, and character strengths in mindfulness-based interventions: A psychological science perspective. *Mindfulness, 6*, 956–969. https://doi.org/10.1007/s12671-015-0419-2

Baxter, H. J., Johnson, M. H., & Bean, D. (2012). Efficacy of a character strengths and gratitude intervention for people with chronic back pain. *The Australian Journal of Rehabilitation Counseling, 18*(2), 135–147. https://doi.org/10.1017/jrc.2012.14

Bertisch, H., Rath, J., Long, C., Ashman, T., & Rashid, T. (2014). Positive psychology in rehabilitation medicine: A brief report. *NeuroRehabilitation, 34*(3), 573–585.

Bretherton, R., & Niemiec, R. M. (2019). Mindfulness-based strengths practice (MBSP). In I. Ivtzan (Ed.), *Handbook of mindfulness-based programmes* (pp. 385–402). Routledge.

Bu, H., & Duan, W. (2021). Strength-based flourishing intervention to promote resilience in individuals with physical disabilities in disadvantaged communities: A randomized controlled trial. *Research on Social Work Practice, 31*(1), 53–64. https://doi-org.ezproxy.cul.columbia.edu/10.1177/1049731520959445

Casali, N., Feraco, T., Ghisi, M., & Meneghetti, C. (2020). "Andrà tutto bene": Associations between character strengths, psychological distress and self-efficacy during covid-19 lockdown. *Journal of Happiness Studies*. Advance online publication. https://doi.org/10.1007/s10902-020-00321-w.

Casali, N., Feraco, T., & Meneghetti, C. (2021). Character strengths sustain mental health and post-traumatic growth during the COVID-19 pandemic. A longitudinal analysis. *Psychology and Health*. https://doi.org/10.1080/08870446.2021.1952587

Chan, K., Wong, F. K., & Lee, P. H. (2019). A brief hope intervention to increase hope level and improve well-being in rehabilitating cancer patients: A feasibility test. *Sage Open Nursing, 5*, 2377960819844381.

Chaput, J. P., McHill, A. W., Cox, R. C., Broussard, J. L., Dutil, C., da Costa, B. G., et al. (2023). The role of insufficient sleep and circadian misalignment in obesity. *Nature Reviews Endocrinology, 19*(2), 82–97.

Chaves, C., Hervas, G., García, F. E., & Vazquez, C. (2016a). Building life satisfaction through well-being dimensions: A longitudinal study in children with a life-threatening illness. *Journal of Happiness Studies, 17*(3), 1051–1067. https://doi.org/10.1007/s10902-015-9631-y

Chaves, C., Vázquez, C., & Hervás, G. (2016b). Positive interventions in seriously-ill children: Effects on well-being after granting a wish. *Journal of Health Psychology, 21*(9), 1870–1883. https://doi.org/10.1177/1359105314567768

Cheavens, J. S., & Guter, M. M. (2018). Hope therapy. In M. W. Gallagher & S. J. Lopez (Eds.), *The Oxford handbook of hope* (pp. 133–142). Oxford University Press.

Datu, J., & Niemiec, R. M. (2023). *Disability: Character strengths, stigma, and acceptance across different disabilities*. Data from 21,800 people, collected on the VIA Institute on Character website.

Datu, J. A. D., Valdez, J. M., McInerney, D. M., & Cayubit, R. F. (2021). The effects of gratitude and kindness on life satisfaction, positive emotions, negative emotions, and COVID-19 anxiety: An online pilot experimental study. *Applied Psychology Health and Well-Being*. https://doi.org/10.1111/aphw.12306

Department of Psychiatry and Behavioral Sciences. (n.d.). *Compassion cultivation training for physicians and psychologists*. Department of Psychiatry and Behavioral Sciences. Retrieved March 4, 2023, from https://med.stanford.edu/psychiatry/education/cme/cct.html

Emmons, R. A., & McCullough, M. E. (2003). Counting blessings versus burdens: An experimental investigation of gratitude and subjective well-being in daily life. *Journal of Personality and Social Psychology, 84*, 377–389.

Ghosh, A., & Deb, A. (2017). Positive psychology interventions for chronic physical illnesses: A systematic review. *Psychological Studies*. https://doi.org/10.1007/s12646-017-0421-y

Graziosi, M., Yaden, D., Clifton, J., Mikanik, N., & Niemiec, R. M. (2020). A strengths-based approach to chronic pain. *Journal of Positive Psychology*. https://doi.org/10.1080/17439760.2020.1858337

Hanks, R. A., Rapport, L. J., Waldron-Perrine, B., & Millis, S. R. (2014). Role of character strengths in outcome after mild complicated to severe traumatic brain injury: A positive psychology study. *Archives of Physical Medicine and Rehabilitation, 95*(11), 2096–2102. https://doi.org/10.1016/j.apmr.2014.06.017

Hausler, M., Strecker, C., Huber, A., Brenner, M., Höge, T., & Höfer, S. (2017). Associations between the application of signature character strengths, health and well-being of health professionals. *Frontiers in Psychology, 8*. https://doi.org/10.3389/fpsyg.2017.01307

Hirsch, J. K., Treaster, M. K., Kaniuka, A. R., Brooks, B. D., Sirois, F. M., Kohls, N., Nöfer, E., Toussaint, L. L., & Offenbächer, M. (2019). Fibromyalgia impact and depressive symptoms: Can perceiving a silver lining make a difference? *Scandinavian Journal of Psychology*. https://doi.org/10.1111/sjop.12598

Höge, T., Strecker, C., Hausler, M., Huber, A., & Höfer, S. (2019). Perceived socio-moral climate and the applicability of signature character strengths at work: A study among hospital physicians. *Applied Research in Quality of Life*. https://doi.org/10.1007/s11482-018-9697-x

Hoge, E. A., Bui, E., Mete, M., Dutton, M. A., Baker, A. W., & Simon, N. M. (2023). Mindfulness-based stress reduction vs escitalopram for the treatment of adults with anxiety disorders: A randomized clinical trial. *JAMA Psychiatry, 80*(1), 13–21.

Huber, A., Strecker, C., Hausler, M., Kachel, T., Höge, T., & Höfer, S. (2019). Possession and applicability of signature character strengths: What is essential for well-being, work engagement, and burnout? *Applied Research in Quality of Life*. https://doi.org/10.1007/s11482-018-9699-8

Huber, A., Strecker, C., Kachel, T., Hoge, T., & Hofer, S. (2020). Character strengths profiles in medical professionals and their impact on well-being. *Frontiers in Psychology*. https://doi.org/10.3389/fpsyg.2020.566728

Huffman, J. C., Mastromauro, C. A., Boehm, J. K., Seabrook, R., Fricchione, G. L., Denninger, J. W., et al. (2011). Development of a positive psychology intervention for patients with acute cardiovascular disease. *Heart International, 6*(2), e14.

Huffman, J. C., Millstein, R. A., Mastromauro, C. A., Moore, S. V., Celano, C. M., Andres Bedoya, C., Suarez, L., Boehm, J. K., & Januzzi, J. L. (2016). A positive psychology intervention for patients with an acute coronary syndrome: Treatment development and proof-of-concept trial. *Journal of Happiness Studies, 17*(5), 1985–2006. https://doi.org/10.1007/s10902-015-9681-1

Johns, G., Samuel, V., Freemantle, L., Lewis, J., & Waddington, L. (2022). The global prevalence of depression and anxiety among doctors during the covid-19 pandemic: Systematic review and meta-analysis. *Journal of Affective Disorders, 298*, 431–441.

Kachel, T., Huber, A., Strecker, C., Hoge, T., & Hofer, S. (2021). Reality meets belief: A mixed methods study on character strengths and well-being of hospital physicians. *Frontiers in Psychology, 12*. https://doi.org/10.3389/fpsyg.2021.547773

Kawashima, M., Uchino, M., & Tsubota, K. (2018). Value of considering psychological strengths in patients with eye pain. *American Journal of Ophthalmology Case Reports, 12*, 91–92. https://doi.org/10.1016/j.ajoc.2018.10.003

Leventhal, K. S., Gillham, J., DeMaria, L., Andrew, G., Peabody, J., & Leventhal, S. (2015). Building psychosocial assets and wellbeing among adolescent girls: A randomized controlled trial. *Journal of Adolescence, 45*, 284–295. https://doi.org/10.1016/j.adolescence.2015.09.011

Leventhal, K. S., DeMaria, L. M., Gillham, J. E., Andrew, G., Peabody, J., & Leventhal, S. M. (2016). A psychosocial resilience curriculum provides the "missing piece" to boost adolescent physical health: A randomized controlled trial of girls first in India. *Social Science & Medicine, 161*, 37–46. https://doi.org/10.1016/j.socscimed.2016.05.004

Liu, Q., & Wang, Z. (2021). Perceived stress of the COVID-19 pandemic and adolescents' depression symptoms: The moderating role of character strengths. *Personality and Individual Differences, 182*, 111062. https://doi.org/10.1016/j.paid.2021.111062

Livneh, H., & Martz, E. (2016). Psychosocial adaptation to disability within the context of positive psychology: Philosophical aspects and historical roots. *Journal of Occupational Rehabilitation, 26*, 13–19.

Long, K. N., Kim, E. S., Chen, Y., Wilson, M. F., Worthington, E. L., Jr., & VanderWeele, T. J. (2020). The role of hope in subsequent health and well-being for older adults: An outcome-wide longitudinal approach. *Global Epidemiology, 2*, 100018.

Lottman, T., Zawaly, S., & Niemiec, R. M. (2017). Well-being and well-doing: Bringing mindfulness and character strengths to the early childhood classroom and home. In C. Proctor (Ed.), *Positive psychology interventions in practice* (pp. 83–105). Springer. https://doi.org/10.1007/978-3-319-51787-2_6

Macfarlane, J. (2019). Exploring how awareness of character strengths can benefit mental health nurses. *British Journal of Mental Health Nursing, 8*(3), 145–152. https://doi.org/10.12968/bjmh.2019.8.3.145

Macfarlane, J. (2022). Positive psychology pioneers: Ryan Niemiec's power and potential to influence mental health nursing. *British Journal of Mental Health Nursing*. https://doi.org/10.12968/bjmh.2022.0032

Martinez-Marti, M. L., Theirs, C. I., Pascual, D., & Corradi, G. (2020). Character strengths predict an increase in mental health and subjective well-being over a one-month period during the COVID-19 pandemic lockdown. *Frontiers in Psychology*. https://doi.org/10.3389/fpsyg.2020.584567

Mayo Foundation for Medical Education and Research. (2022a, November 1). *5 basics of a well-rounded fitness routine*. Mayo Clinic. Retrieved March 4, 2023, from https://www.mayoclinic.org/healthy-lifestyle/fitness/in-depth/fitness-training/art-20044792

Mayo Foundation for Medical Education and Research. (2022b, May 7). *6 steps to better sleep*. Mayo Clinic. Retrieved March 4, 2023, from https://www.mayoclinic.org/healthy-lifestyle/adult-health/in-depth/sleep/art-20048379

Monzani, L., Escartin, J., Ceja, L., & Bakker, A. B. (2021). Blending mindfulness practices and character strengths increases employee wellbeing: A second-order meta-analysis and a follow-up field experiment. *Human Resource Management Journal*. https://doi.org/10.1111/1748-8583.12360

Niemiec, R. M. (2012). Mindful living: Character strengths interventions as pathways for the five mindfulness trainings. *International Journal of Wellbeing, 2*(1), 22–33. https://doi.org/10.5502/ijw.v2i1.2

Niemiec, R. M. (2018). *Character strengths interventions: A field-guide for practitioners*. Hogrefe.

Niemiec, R. M. (2019a). Six functions of character strengths for thriving at times of adversity and opportunity: A theoretical perspective. *Applied Research in Quality of Life*. https://doi.org/10.1007/s11482-018-9692-2. Full PDF Article

Niemiec, R. M. (2019b). *The strengths-based workbook for stress relief*. New Harbinger.

Niemiec, R. M. (2023). Mental health and character strengths: The dual-role of boosting well-being and reducing suffering. *Mental Health and Social Inclusion*. https://doi.org/10.1108/MHSI-01-2023-0012

Niemiec, R. M., & Yarova, A. (2018). Character strengths and health: Research summary (part 1). *Chronicle of Advances in Positive Health and Well-being, 1*(1) Available at: http://www.ippanetwork.org/positive-health/character-strengths-and-health-research-summary-part-1/

Pang, D., & Ruch, W. (2019). Fusing character strengths and mindfulness interventions: Benefits for job satisfaction and performance. *Journal of Occupational Health Psychology, 24*(1), 150–162. https://doi.org/10.1037/ocp0000144

Peterson, C., Park, N., & Seligman, M. E. P. (2006). Greater strengths of character and recovery from illness. *The Journal of Positive Psychology, 1*(1), 17–26.

Proyer, R. T., Gander, F., Wellenzohn, S., & Ruch, W. (2013). What good are character strengths beyond subjective well-being? The contribution of the good character on self-reported health-oriented behavior, physical fitness, and the subjective health status. *Journal of Positive Psychology*.

Rashid, T., & McGrath, R. E. (2020). Strengths-based actions to enhance wellbeing in the time of COVID19. *International Journal of Wellbeing, 10*(4), 113–132. https://doi.org/10.5502/ijw.v10i4.1441

Reycraft, J. T., Islam, H., Townsend, L. K., Hayward, G. C., Hazell, T. J., & Macpherson, R. E. K. (2020). Exercise intensity and recovery on circulating brain-derived neurotrophic factor. *Med Sci Sports Exercise, 52*(5), 1210–1217. https://doi.org/10.1249/MSS.0000000000002242

Seligman, M. E. P. (2008). Positive health. *Applied Psychology, 57*(1), 3–18. https://doi.org/10.1111/j.1464-0597.2008.00351.x

Seoane, L., Tompkins, L. M., De Conciliis, A., & Boysen, P. G. (2016). Virtues education in medical school: The foundation for professional formation. *The Ochsner Journal, 16*(1), 50–55.

Shinichiro, M., Kawashima, M., Uchino, M., & Tsubota, K. (2018). Value of considering psychological strengths in patients with eye pain. *American Journal of Ophthalmology Case Reports, 12*, 91–92. https://doi.org/10.1016/j.ajoc.2018.10.003

Shogren, K. A., Singh, N., Niemiec, R. M., & Wehmeyer, M. (2017). Character strengths and mindfulness. In M. Wehmeyer (Ed.), *Oxford handbooks online*. https://doi.org/10.1093/oxfordhb/9780199935291.013.77

Smedema, S. M. (2020). An analysis of the relationship of character strengths and quality of life in persons with multiple sclerosis. *Quality of Life Research*. https://doi.org/10.1007/s11136-019-02397-1

Snyder, C. R., Harris, C., Anderson, J. R., Holleran, S. A., Irving, L. M., Sigmon, S. T., Yoshinobu, L., Gibb, J., Langelle, C., & Harney, P. (1991). The will and the ways: Development and validation of an individual-differences measure of hope. *Journal of Personality and Social Psychology, 60*(4), 570–585. https://doi.org/10.1037/0022-3514.60.4.570

Strecker, C., Huber, A., Höge, T., Hausler, M., & Höfer, S. (2019). Identifying thriving workplaces in hospitals: Work characteristics and the applicability of character strengths at work. *Applied Research in Quality of Life*. https://doi.org/10.1007/s11482-018-9693-1

Stuntz, C. P. (2018). Differences in character strengths levels and associations with positive outcomes across contexts. *Journal of Positive Psychology and Wellbeing, 3*(1), 45–61.

Szuhany, K. L., Malgaroli, M., & Bonanno, G. A. (2023). Physical activity may buffer against depression and promote resilience after major life stressors. *Mental Health and Physical Activity, 24*, 100505.

Tang, Y. Y., Posner, M. I., & Rothbart, M. K. (2014). Meditation improves self-regulation over the life span. *Annals of the New York Academy of Sciences, 1307*(1), 104–111.

Tomasulo, D. (2020). *Learned hopefulness: The power of positivity to overcome depression*. New Harbinger.

Trzeciak, S., Roberts, B. W., & Mazzarelli, A. J. (2017). Compassionomics: Hypothesis and experimental approach. *Medical Hypotheses, 107*, 92–97.

Umucu, E., Tansey, T. N., Brooks, J., & Lee, B. (2020). The protective role of character strengths in COVID-19 stress and well-being in individuals with chronic conditions and disabilities: An exploratory study. *Rehabilitation Counseling Bulletin*. https://doi.org/10.1177/0034355220967093

VanderWeele, T. J. (2019). Reimagining health – Flourishing. *Journal of the American Medical Association (JAMA)*, E1–E2. https://doi.org/10.1001/jama.2019.3035

Vasileiou, D., Moraitou, D., Papaliagkas, V., Pezirkianidis, C., Stalikas, A., Papantoniou, G., & Sofologi, M. (2021). The relationships between character strengths and subjective wellbeing: Evidence from Greece under lockdown during COVID-19 pandemic. *International Journal of Environmental Research and Public Health, 18*.

Waters, L., Algoe, S. B., Dutton, J., Emmons, R., Fredrickson, B. L., Heaphy, E., Moskowitz, J. T., Neff, K., Niemiec, R. M., Pury, C., & Steger, M. (2021). Positive psychology in a pandemic: Buffering, bolstering, and building mental health. *Journal of Positive Psychology*. https://doi.org/10.1080/17439760.2021.1871945

West, C. P., Dyrbye, L. N., Erwin, P. J., & Shanafelt, T. D. (2016). Interventions to prevent and reduce physician burnout: A systematic review and meta-analysis. *The Lancet, 388*(10057), 2272–2281.

Weziak-Bialowolska, D., Bialowolski, P., & Niemiec, R. M. (2021). Being good, doing good: The role of honesty and integrity for health. *Social Science and Medicine, 291*. https://doi.org/10.1016/j.socscimed.2021.114494

Weziak-Bialowolska, D., Bialowolski, P., & Niemiec, R. M. (2023). Character strengths and health-related quality of life in a large international sample: A cross-sectional analysis. *Journal of Research in Personality, 103*. https://doi.org/10.1016/j.jrp.2022.104338

Whelan-Berry, K., & Niemiec, R. M. (2021). Integrating mindfulness and character strengths for improved well-being, stress, and relationships: A qualitative analysis of mindfulness-based strengths practice. *International Journal of Wellbeing, 11*(2). https://doi.org/10.5502/ijw.v11i2.1545

Wingert, J. R., Jones, J. C., Swoap, R. A., & Wingert, H. M. (2020). Mindfulness-based strengths practice improves well-being and retention in undergraduates: A preliminary randomized controlled trial. *Journal of American College Health*. Advance Online Publication. https://doi.org/10.1080/07448481.2020.1764005.

Yan, T., Chan, C. W. H., Chow, K. M., Zheng, W., & Sun, M. (2020). A systematic review of the effects of character strengths-based intervention on the psychological well-being of patients suffering from chronic illnesses. *Journal of Advanced Nursing, 76*(7), 1567–1580. https://doi.org/10.1111/jan.14356

Part III
Special Topics for Intellectual/Developmental Disabilities and Character Strengths

The chapters in this section target the population of people with different kinds of intellectual/developmental disabilities and the people who support, treat, and/or care for them.

The special topics include dual-diagnosis (Chap. 8), the work of justice, equity, diversity, inclusion (JEDI; Chap. 9), and the integration of spirituality and meaning (Chap. 10). These chapters continue the structure of focusing on the central concepts within each area and how character strengths inform, enhance, or integrate with the topic. This is followed by a review of the scientific studies relating to each topic and a discussion of core character strengths practices to bring benefit to that area for people with intellectual/developmental disability.

Chapter 8
Dual Diagnosis and Character Strengths

Our lives begin to end the day we become silent about things that matter.

–Dr. Martin Luther King Jr

The Concepts

Dual diagnosis (DD) is the coexistence of intellectual/developmental disability (IDD) and at least one psychiatric disorder (Werner & Stawski, 2012). Note that dual diagnosis can sometimes be confused to mean the coexistence of substance abuse and mental illness. It is estimated that between 1% and 2% of the world's population has IDD and that the prevalence rate is twice as high in low and middle-income countries (Maulik et al., 2011). For people with IDD, mental illness happens much more often than in the general population (McConkey et al., 2019).

For comparison, the incidence of a mental health disorder in the general population is estimated at approximately 10% (Dattani et al., 2021). In conflict-affected populations (countries with major conflict-induced humanitarian crises), this number more than doubles to 22% (Charlson et al., 2019). Yet, when compared to the general population, people with an IDD have more than triple the prevalence rate at 33% (Mazza et al., 2020). For children with IDD, the situation is even worse. In a recent study, the pooled prevalence estimate is 38% (Buckley et al., 2020).

The current edition of *Intellectual and Developmental Disabilities: Definition, Diagnosis, Classification, and Planning Supports* (12th ed.) by the American Association on Intellectual and Developmental Disabilities (AAIDD), the leading authority on Intellectual and Developmental Disability, defines an IDD as "…significant limitations in both intellectual functioning and adaptive behavior as expressed in conceptual, social, and practical skills" (p. 51). Based on recent studies of brain development, IDD is identified as originating during a developmental period before the person reaches the age of 22 (Schalock et al., 2021).

People with IDD have been and continue to be discriminated against, locked away, and even killed (Reinders et al., 2019). Since the mid-1800s, there have been shifting approaches to the treatment and care for people with an IDD that began with optimism but shifted to a need to protect individuals with IDD, then an attitude

R. M. Niemiec, D. Tomasulo, *Character Strengths and Abilities Within Disabilities*, Positive Psychology and Disability Series,
https://doi.org/10.1007/978-3-031-36294-1_8

and treatment shift to protect society from people with IDD (Ilyes, 2020). This shifting emphasis from optimism to the protection of the individual, to the protection of society has been a setback in developing psychological, educational, and behavioral technology. When the goal is to protect society, such as in the case of criminals and the use of prisons, the approach is to restrict, contain, limit, and monitor. For people with IDD, this meant being institutionalized and kept from society with no opportunity or plan for improving one's conditions (Tomasulo, 2018). There was no notion of rehabilitation—or, more accurately, habilitation-and no interest in supporting mental health needs. People placed in institutions were "put away." Indeed, the generic term for those with IDD in institutions was "incurables." This term defined both attitude and effort put into treatment.

As medical labels changed from idiot, imbecile, moron, and feeblemindedness, attitudes toward the "incurables" changed—and along with this, so did the approach to more humanized treatment (Herat, 2021). Yet, while there has been significant progress, it is important to know that the field of IDD, because of these earlier labels and prevailing attitudes, has a long and tragic history (Guercio, 2020). It is filled with neglect and atrocities. Not the least of which is the 20-year legal battle of the infamous Willowbrook school on Staten Island, one of the most notorious institutions in the United States.

In 1972, television journalist Geraldo Rivera illegally filmed the intellectually disabled inmates at Willowbrook in their squalor. This became a turning point for the treatment and care of people with IDD. Within 10 min, Rivera and his crew were in and out with the footage, and the videos were aired on the New York Channel 7 news. The atrocities captured by the images created a public outcry igniting the legal system.

This was the tipping point in US history when mental health treatment became a civil right. Before Willowbrook, institutions served the misguided notion that society must be protected. The result was the height of institutional prejudice and abuse as individuals were at the mercy of the authorities. Protection for the most vulnerable among us was not a consideration. But crucially, the legal battles paid off. The news reports became the impetus for the Willowbrook Consent Decree, a major contributing factor to the passage of the Civil Rights of Institutionalized Persons Act of 1980. Now, every individual in an institution, be it a prison or nursing home, group home, or residential facility has a right to treatment for their mental health.

This legal turning point in treatment and care for individuals with IDD was ushered in through a psychological emphasis on behavioral management and applying behavioral principles. As this approach gained favor, research was mounting that could demonstrate negative or unwanted behaviors, and desirable or adaptive behaviors could be modified through the principles of reinforcement and punishment (Guercio, 2020). Despite these efforts, the field since 1980 has largely been dominated by a focus on ameliorating deficit behaviors, not cultivating strengths.

While things have slowly changed and are emerging for the better, discrimination against people with IDD is still a major problem in many parts of the world (Scior, et al., 2020). The current emphasis from AAIDD and other professional agencies is on emphasizing quality of life for individuals with IDD as a primary emphasis of treatment and measurement (Brown et al., 2022). The problem is that the mental health needs of people with IDD, while more than three times higher than the general population (Mazza et al., 2020), are not being adequately addressed. Importantly, it is the attitude of professionals toward treatment and measurement approaches that is central to success. Toward this end, using character strengths in vocational, educational, and clinical practices is becoming a major tool for facilitating quality-of-life initiatives that directly address mental health needs. As this happens, it will continue to enhance self-esteem for people with IDD (Schwartz et al. 2022).

The AAIDD has set the standard for treatment by using five essential assumptions for applying their definition (Schaloc et al., 2021). These are instructive, and #3 (italics added) is particularly important for this chapter.

1. Limitations in present functioning must be considered within the context of community environments typical of the individual's age, peers, and culture.
2. Valid assessment considers cultural and linguistic diversity as well as differences in communication, sensory, motor, and behavioral factors.
3. *Within an individual, limitations often co-exist with strengths.*
4. An important purpose of describing limitations is to develop a profile of needed supports.
5. With appropriate personalized supports over a sustained period, the life functioning of the person with ID generally will improve.

"*Within an individual, limitations often co-exist with strengths.*" This simple but profound assumption is more than an acknowledgment of the existence of strengths that may have been eclipsed by the limitation imposed by an IDD. Rather, it is a call to action for researchers and practitioners to understand that these unique strengths exist within individuals with dual diagnoses, to search for, identify, and nurture them, and then honor and celebrate their emergence regularly. It is the co-occurrence of strengths, in particular, character strengths, that will enhance the practitioner's approach to treating the impact of the disabilities. The strategic stance for practitioners is to acknowledge the limitations of an IDD while providing support and guidance in helping to develop character. In this way those with an IDD can find ways to thrive, and those with a dual diagnosis can have the advantage of reducing the suffering that comes from coping with a mental illness, while increasing well-being.

Professional responsibilities for those working with IDD include the typical building blocks of relationships, such as respect for the person and practicing professional ethics and standards in applying clinical judgment. The professional practices include using evidence-based practices that get evaluated in a person-centered way for individual benefit and societal enhancement (Luckasson et al., 2022). Toward this end, integrating character strengths as a vehicle for cultivating relationships, increasing positive experiences, and facilitating accomplishments seems tailor-made for implementation with people with IDD. Character strength interventions are evidence-based and person-centered, with individual and societal gains. By considering character as a worthy pursuit to develop, the emphasis is not to replace gains made through behavior modification and applied behavior analysis

(ABA). Rather, character development is an additive approach to treatment. Treatment of the whole person, of behavioral and characterological expressions together, will help ensure that the gains made are sustained.

The Science

The Willowbrook State School was finally shuttered in 1987 following public outcry over its deplorable conditions. But in its wake was left the very real difficulty of attempting to do research on people with IDD (Iacono, 2006). While the conditions at Willowbrook were horrific, the most egregious had to do with scientists obtaining institutional and parental permission and then conducting research and doing the unthinkable. Children with IDD were infected with viral hepatitis without their knowledge. More than this, the informed consent obtained from their parents was questionable and may have been coerced.

In the shadow of the Willowbrook, Institutional Review Boards (IRBs—the governing bodies of institutions that allow for human research to be conducted) tend to err on the side of being too conservative and overregulate (Aman & Handen, 2006). As a result, it is more difficult to conduct research that includes people with IDD (Iacono, 2006). While guarding against potential exploitation and harm, the rights of people with IDD to be included in research related to their well-being must be honored. While efforts to evolve how IRBs function and approve research have been proposed, the reality remains that the volume of research on people with IDD in a clinical setting is much less than is needed. In an article by Vereenooghe et al. (2018), the researchers retrieved 41,232 records and of those reviewed 573 full-text articles. This was in an effort to identify *interventions for mental health problems in children and adults with severe IDD. They found three pharmacological studies* and only two studies evaluating psychological interventions. Their conclusion was that the evidence is too limited to identify effective treatments for people with IDD. The statistic of two articles out of 573 unveils the difficulty of getting research approved and yielding sufficient outcomes to lead to practical interventions for improving mental health. This means evidence-based interventions need to be supplemented with evidence-informed approaches. Research effective with other populations must be extrapolated, and creative ways of adapting what is known to work with others are being applied to people with IDD. In this context, there are several applied approaches being employed, and many of them involve the application of evidence-informed use of character strengths (Niemiec et al. 2017; Shogren et al., 2017).

What was learned from Willowbrook is that when people are given a chance to feel safe and the opportunity to learn, they can thrive. Once given the safety and opportunity to learn, then the tools used to help this learning take place are key. The advent of the science of character strengths nearly 20 years ago is a turning point in the history of psychology (Peterson & Seligman, 2004), which simultaneously signaled a turning point in the stance taken by psychologists toward the treatment of IDD (Niemiec et al., 2017).

By shifting away from IQ as the primary measure and prediction of success and focusing on what is strong rather than what is wrong with an individual, the emphasis on psychology as a science and practice evolved radically. Historically, psychological research and practice focused on the identification of pathology and the amelioration of suffering. But this has failed to yield significant progress in helping people sustain changes in their well-being (Seligman, 2002).

Within the field of IDD, it opened up a way of thinking about the whole person—not just the person presenting behavioral and psychological difficulties. It provided tools to measure positive, non-intellectually related components of one's individuality. Rather than being defined by a single IQ score, people with an IDD could be viewed holistically. Their limitations, which were able to be thoroughly identified and quantified, could now be seen as coexisting with equally recognizable and measurable traits and assets rather than faults. Indeed, Binet's original hope was for his IQ assessment to be used to understand the strengths of children better and build curricula around it (Ilyes, 2020). Perhaps character development is a return to that intent. If Willowbrook ended the institutional era for intellectually disabled citizens, perhaps character strengths will end the reign of IQ as the measure of an individual.

In a recent assessment of clinicians using the VIA Survey with individuals with intellectual and/or developmental disabilities, it was found that introducing and discussing these strengths led to a framework for self-knowledge, self-understanding, and self-esteem (Schwartz et al., 2022). This is promising and suggests that the survey be more accessible to people with IDD. As it is now, third parties fill out the survey based on their observation. Since reading is a currently required skill to fill out the survey, and many people with IDD have no or low literacy, adaptive versions and other measurement approaches are needed (see Chap. 3 for measurement strategies and examples for people with IDD).

As with other research in the history of psychology, the literature and emphasis on people with IDD have focused on deficits, impairment, and problematic concerns. Added to this is the issue of inadequate research which suggests that focusing on the problems alone does not yield much useful information. As the science pivots, this becomes the moment in history when an explicit focus on the intersection of positive psychology and IDD needs to be emphasized, highlighted, and cultivated. The understanding, measurement, and facilitation of character strengths provides the framework for such reformation, representation, and realization.

Although still small in number, a systematic review of the literature between 1992 and 2019 assessed positive psychological constructs in samples that included individuals with IDD. It was found that a total of 16 studies used 22 different measures testing more than a dozen positive psychology constructs. Chief among these were character strengths which yielded positive emotional well-being and growth (Albaum et al., 2021).

Finding the path to creating optimal functioning for individuals with IDD will rely heavily on assumptions put forth by the AAIDD. In particular, researchers and practitioners must continue to find ways to address the limitations while searching for coexisting strengths by developing measurement tools (Raley et al., 2020) and effective strengths-based interventions. Furthermore, the rationale for implementing a strength-based perspective goes beyond helping individuals with IDD. It has implications for families and those who provide support.

The United Nations Convention on the Rights of Persons with a Disability declared the emphasis should be on transforming services from institutional to community-based programs and initiatives (UN General Assembly, 2006). This effort continues and is designed to both reduce costs while increasing well-being, and there is evidence that suggests both are possible. In an intriguing way, this means that as less money and resources are being spent, a higher quality of life is possible. How can this be? Specifically, people with IDD receiving consistently good active support experienced a better quality of life. Strengths-based measures of emotional well-being, personal development, interpersonal relationships, social inclusion, and self-determination have validated this. When staff are actively supportive and interactive, they offer good support without investing more time or higher costs (Beadles-Brown et al., 2021). Other researchers determined that promoting a mindfulness practice (which is a strengths-based approach) for support providers helps to change the support relationship to one that is strengths-based (Singh et al., 2009). When providers in the community are oriented in a strength-based fashion and offer active support, the outcome will likely be a higher quality of life for all at less cost. A strength-based approach is both psychologically advantageous and cost-effective.

Additional scientific studies are embedded in the subsequent section on practice to better align with the concepts and discussion therein.

The Practice

The use of character strengths has important implications for improving the lives of people with IDD. The areas we discuss in this section seem to have the greatest potential for applying character strengths. The areas of employment, education, and therapy have seen important gains in the general population, and we believe that with modifications, they will be the arenas where progress will occur.

At a societal level, the reason why employment is so important is that an individual who is gainfully employed adds to the productivity of the workforce while paying taxes that go back to support society. This is why there are incentives for employers to work with disabled individuals and why there are many government-supported agencies to help educate and train people with disabilities looking to enter the workforce. At a personal level, typically, in the general population, when you are employed you will have a higher quality of life and better mental health. There is also some evidence that if you are intellectually disabled and are working this is true as well (Dean et al., 2018).

There is a mindset that with the habilitation of people with IDD that, at some point, they may or do become employable. While this may not be the goal for those with severe and profound levels of IDD, it is a goal that most agencies and community-based programs have as an aspiration. Yet, despite this pervasive objective, people with IDD typically experience low rates of paid employment—even though they can make important, valuable contributions to the workplace (Lysaght et al., 2012). At a practical level, one research study on the typical population showed that a job search that includes the understanding and use of character strengths led to increased employment rates (80%) compared to traditional career counseling (60%) (Littman-Ovadia, et al., 2014). Character strengths have also been found to facilitate job satisfaction and feeling one's work is a calling in life, especially when the person reports using multiple top signature strengths at work (Harzer & Ruch, 2015). If we extrapolate from the research, people with IDD and a mental illness who learn to use their signature strengths may be more employable, have greater job satisfaction, have a higher quality of life, and better mental health. They will also have the dignity that comes from making their own money and contributing back to the community through taxes.

In addition to character strengths applications in the workplace, the application of character strengths in education for people with dual diagnosis is also centrally important. The addition of character strengths in education has the potential to amplify and extend the outcomes offered by behavioral management and adaptive behavioral strategies, to improve well-being and, ultimately, quality of life. This has been the case when character education was added to curriculums for non-disabled students and seems likely to have a similar impact for students with dual-diagnosis (Yin & Majid, 2018).

Specific to dual diagnosis, people with IDD have greater clinical needs due to a higher likelihood of having a secondary psychological disorder (Vereenooghe et al., 2018), but this is rarely perceived or acknowledged, largely due to a phenomenon known as "diagnostic overshadowing" (Reiss et al., 1982). This term reflects the tendency of clinicians to use the umbrella of IDD to subsume various psychopathologies. This causes an emotional issue, and even one as common as grieving, to remain unchecked, naturally resulting in the condition going untreated. In the American Psychological Association's *Guidelines for Assessment of and Intervention with Persons with Disabilities* (American Psychological Association, APA Task Force on Guidelines for Assessment and Intervention with Persons with Disabilities, 2022), "diagnostic overshadowing" is identified more broadly as a continuing obstruction in treating any person with a disability. Such a perspective ignores other important aspects of the person's life, such as life events, capabilities, and strengths. This is particularly pertinent regarding therapy for people with IDD. It means psychologists are not going to look for, perceive, understand, or consequently treat someone who has a primary IDD. The APA itself points to a lack of preparation for psychologists as the problem (American Psychological Association, APA Task Force on Guidelines for Assessment and Intervention with Persons with Disabilities, 2022).

> Unfortunately, while psychologists receive extensive training in how to approach mental health issues, they rarely receive adequate education or training in disability. Few graduate psychology training programs offer disability coursework. Limited training and experience may leave many psychologists unprepared to provide professionally and ethically sound services to clients with disabilities. Further, many psychologists seek to develop disability competence after they have completed formal training (p. 2).

One step toward the amelioration of this gap in training is the creation of the *Diagnostic Manual for People with IDD* (DM-ID 2) (Fletcher et al., 2017). This evidence-based manual highlights the shift in diagnostic criteria used for people with IDD. As an example, the usual symptoms of Post-traumatic Stress Disorder (PTSD) in a non-ID population require that the individual has been exposed to a traumatic event where the person experienced, witnessed, or was confronted with an event or events that involved actual or threatened death or serious injury, or a threat to the physical integrity of self or others But what constitutes the activation of a traumatic reaction in a non-ID population may be vastly different for someone with limited cognitive abilities. According to the DM-ID:

"In assessing for traumatic exposure in people with ID, take note that events such as developmental milestones, residential placement, and even adult, consensual sexual experiences have led to posttraumatic reactions in some individuals with ID. It appears that the range of potentially traumatizing events is greater for individuals with a lower developmental age…" (p. 373).

Promoting greater interest and awareness about the needs of people with IDD and efforts to see beyond overshadowing does not relieve the issue of people with IDD being excluded from studies mentioned earlier. More awareness needs to be coupled with more research. Even if the primary IDD no longer eclipses the clinical picture, a more accurate understanding of the differences in how symptoms and conditions might manifest will be needed.

IBT and P-IBT[1]

Adapting evidence-informed interventions to more accurately meet the clinical needs is necessary. In this vein, one of the authors (DT) developed Interactive-Behavioral Therapy (IBT) and later Positive-Interactive Behavioral therapy (P-IBT). Both are modified forms of group psychotherapy shown to be effective with people with dual diagnosis. Highlights of this model drawn from the literature are offered (Tomasulo, 2014).

IBT has been the subject of a number of studies and the subject of the American Psychological Association's first book on psychotherapy for people with IDD (Razza & Tomasulo, 2005). The aim of IBT was to use a remodeled group format to generate the same therapeutic gain for adults with an ID that was available to the general population. The adapted model focused on activation of therapeutic factors. Therapeutic factors are those features of a group process that have therapeutic value for members and are identified as: acceptance/cohesion; universality; altruism; instillation of hope; guidance; vicarious learning/modeling; catharsis; imparting of information; self-disclosure; self-understanding; interpersonal learning; corrective

[1] An earlier version of portions of the material from the section on IBT and P-IBT was previously published in an article Tomasulo, D. J. (2014). Positive group psychotherapy modified for adults with IDD. *Journal of IDD*, *18*(4), 337–350.

recapitulation of the primary family; development of socializing techniques; existential factors. These factors have been written about extensively elsewhere and the reader is directed to these sources for more information (e.g., Tomasulo, 2014).

The IBT model uses a role-playing format to activate therapeutic factors that emerge naturally within a group. Specific techniques, such as the empty chair, doubling, and role reversal, are used to engage members in situations where they can both give and receive. The accumulated result of these efforts, as noted by the research below, results in greater well-being for the members by activating therapeutic factors. In recent years the effective use of character strengths with positive psychotherapy (Rashid, 2020; Rashid & Seligman, 2018) has been incorporated into the IBT model, which has been renamed to Positive-Interactive Behavioral Therapy (P-IBT). Facilitators are now trained to not only notice the original 14 therapeutic factors but also the 24 character strengths as they emerge from individual members. P-IBT strengthens group dynamics through interactive role-playing, which elicits therapeutic factors, and individual character strength activation through strength-spotting done by facilitators and group members as well.

A study in positive psychotherapy conducted in a group therapy format will highlight implications for P-IBT. Forty mild to moderately depressed University of Pennsylvania students were divided into a treatment and a non-treatment group. The treatment condition consisted of two groups of 8–11 participants seen for 6 weeks for 2-h sessions. The session was half a discussion of the exercise assigned from the previous week and an introduction to the new exercise. The participants completed homework assignments and reported back each week on their progress. In the first week participants were asked to take the VIA Survey and use their top five strengths more often in their daily lives. Week two involved writing down three good things that had happened during the day and why one believes they occurred. During the third week, participants were asked to write a brief essay on what they, themselves, wanted to be remembered for the most, that is, a biography of having lived a satisfying life. The next session involved composing a letter of gratitude to someone they may never have thanked adequately and reading it to them in person or by phone. During the fifth session, the members were asked to respond very positively and enthusiastically each day to good news received by someone else. The final session involved savoring daily events in their lives that they normally did not take the time to enjoy, and journaling how this experience differed from their normally rushed occurrence. Time was also spent during this last session on tailoring the exercises for their use following the end of the study.

The group PPT participants did better than the no-treatment group on assessments of depression and satisfaction with life. But there is a powerful finding beyond this positive change. The gains made by the PPT groups were maintained with no other intervention by the researchers throughout a 1-year follow-up. In contrast, the baseline levels of depression for the non-treatment group remained unchanged.

This was six sessions and 12 h, with no booster sessions during the year. This is very unusual in the study of depression and highlights how the use of these exercises involved self-maintaining features that served the participants beyond the intervention. But a closer look at this research shows that while the effects of positive interventions were powerful, they required the participants to be able to read and write. The question becomes: Is it possible to generalize and then modify from these interventions ways in which people with dual diagnosis—some who cannot read and write—can profit from modified interventions?

P-IBT model uses a 4-stage format that is process- rather than content-oriented. The facilitation of the process involves the facilitator(s) guiding the members through each stage: orientation, warm-up and sharing, enactment, and affirmation. Each stage was designed to deepen the group's viability by using methods to stimulate the emergence of behaviors related to a particular therapeutic factor or character strength and acknowledging it. As part of their training, facilitators were shown videotapes of how therapeutic factors and character strengths emerge within a P-IBT group and instructed on how to prepare for and acknowledge them.

The orientation stage uses a technique dubbed "cognitive networking" to allow members to get ready for the group process by listening and feeding back what they heard. The topic of discussion during this initial stage is not as important as the process. Members are invited to speak and listen as a way of getting ready to participate. The primary intellectual and psychopathology difficulties and secondary disabilities (such as audiological, visual, and attentional deficits) necessitated a preliminary stage to help participants orient to the group.

The warm-up and sharing stage is designed to help move members from horizontal self-disclosure (disclosure about the act of disclosure itself) toward vertical disclosure (in-depth disclosure about the content). In people with an IDD the horizontal self-disclosure might take the form of saying: "Something happened at the bus stop yesterday." The vertical disclosure might be: "I was called a retard, and the person laughed at me and made me feel terrible."

The enactment stage uses action methods from the field of psychodrama to role-play emotionally salient scenes from a chosen protagonist, which becomes the focus of the group's work for the day. The three techniques used are the empty chair, doubling, and role reversal.

The empty chair is a classic version of the technique originally developed by psychodrama founder Jacob Moreno (Giacomucci, 2021). The protagonist engages with an empty chair representing another person, a future or past self, or another entity.

With doubling, the protagonist is invited to express feelings evoked by an interpersonal situation while the group members listen. The membership is then asked to stand behind (if this is agreeable to the protagonist) or alongside and represent and establish identity with the protagonist by verbalizing what the protagonist is feeling. The accuracy or alignment of these feeling statements with the protagonist is confirmed or corrected with help from the facilitator(s). In multiple doubling, more than one group participant is asked to identify with the protagonist. This creates multiple perspectives for both the protagonist and other group members and provides the protagonist with the feeling of being understood and supported, and typically fosters the therapeutic factors of cohesion, universality, altruism, hope, guidance, vicarious learning, imparting of information, self-disclosure, self-understanding, interpersonal learning, development of socializing techniques and integration. The normal egocentric nature of individuals with ID and concomitant psychopathology is lessened by the protagonist listening for the accuracy of the double and by having those doubling attempt empathic understanding for the protagonist.

Finally, the role reversal technique provides role clarification, reality testing, and most important, empathic development as the protagonist is asked to "step into another's shoes." Once the enactment is completed, and if time permits, others in the group may take their turn as the protagonist.

Throughout the first three stages, incidents of therapeutic factors and character strengths that have occurred within the group are acknowledged by the facilitators. Simple acts of moving a chair to allow someone to enter the group (altruism/kindness); and spontaneous comments such as: "You're going to be all right" (instillation of hope/love), or "I felt like that, too," (universality), are recognized and affirmed by the facilitators.

The affirmation stage allows for the facilitators to review therapeutic factors and character strengths that have emerged throughout the group and relay these instances back to each member. Over time the members are taught to give feedback to one another during this phase, which also allowed for positive emotional closure of each session.

Perhaps the most important intervention involves identifying character strengths before each P- IBT group begins. Flückiger and his colleagues (Flückiger & Grosse Holtforth, 2008) have developed a procedure called resource priming in which the facilitators of psychotherapy take a few minutes before their session to focus on the strengths of their individual client. The result is that the priming leads to resource activation whereby participants focus on the positive perspective of their behavior, which in turn leads to better progress in therapy as measured by a greater reduction in symptoms and higher levels of well-being. Such resource priming is now part of what P-IBT facilitators focus on prior to the group beginning, along with therapeutic factors.

Efficacy of the Model

Although the number of studies is small, the positive findings are encouraging. In one study, researchers tested the efficacy of an IBT group treating both intellectually disabled and non-disabled participants over 17 sessions. Using several measures, it was concluded that both types of patients showed a significant positive change from the therapy, and interestingly, those subjects with IDD demonstrated *higher* frequencies of most therapeutic factors. In addition, each patient set goals and then self-evaluated their success. Final evaluations suggested that patients' achievements of their interpersonal goals in therapy exceeded their expectations (Blaine, 1993). Other researchers confirmed that IBT encouraged the emergence of therapeutic factors (Keller, 1995), and it has also been shown to be effective for dual-diagnosis. In this latter study, 16 weekly sessions of the IBT model were compared to a waiting list with a group of chronically mentally ill adults carrying the diagnosis of schizophrenia or schizoaffective disorder. Multiple clinical rating scales were administered to measure changes in social functioning and negative symptomatology. It was found that: (1) IBT increases the overall social competence of people with chronic schizophrenia or schizoaffective disorders; (2) IBT improves the negative symptoms that are often associated with poor treatment outcomes for people with this diagnosis; and (3) IBT facilitates the emergence of those therapeutic factors found to enhance social competence (Daniels, 1998).

What is of particular interest is that in 16 weeks of treatment with IBT, the *Global Assessment of Functioning Scale*, a scale previously used to assess overall psychosocial functioning and symptom level (see American Psychiatric Association: *Diagnostic and Statistical Manual of Mental Disorders, Fourth Edition, Text Revision* (DSM-IV-TR, 2000)), was significantly improved for the treatment groups. This suggests that the IBT format, in addition to facilitating therapeutic factors, supports the evolution of global social competence. Rather than strengthening behavioral components alone, as would be the goal of an applied behavior analysis approach, the original IBT model yielded a more broad-ranged development of interpersonal socialization.

The IBT model also explored its value in helping individuals with IDD cope with bereavement (Carlin, 1998). Studies have also demonstrated its effectiveness when used concomitantly with behavior modification techniques in treating subjects with both intellectual and psychiatric disorders (Oliver-Brannon, 2000). This later study suffers from a small sample size and non-random assignment. Still, data collection revealed that subjects in the IBT group, compared with the behavior modification controls, evidenced a greater reduction in target behaviors, increased problem-solving skills, and earlier return to the community, further supporting the emphasis on greater global social competence.

In an intriguing pilot study (Lundrigan, 2007), a questionnaire was developed for individuals with IDD based upon Seligman's *Consumer Reports* survey of client satisfaction with mental health services (Seligman, 1995). Although there were only 40 participants in the study, the results are informative about how therapy helps ID participants and how it is perceived. Because most of the participants could not read, researchers administered the survey via a semi-structured interview to 40 IBT participants, all of whom had a psychiatric diagnosis as well as with IQs between 50 and 70. Participants reported feeling helped by their participation in IBT groups, as evidenced by their responses to these questionnaires, and several participants were chosen for in-depth clinical interviews. Of the 40 clients who were surveyed, 34 (85%) felt that they had been helped by participation in an IBT group. It is of note that this figure corresponds closely to the 87% satisfaction rate found in Seligman's *Consumer Reports* study. The high degree of satisfaction reported in the questionnaire further supports the presence of the therapeutic factors in IBT groups reported by other researchers.

The participants entering this study also identified their reasons for treatment. In descending order, the symptoms bringing them for therapy are noted as depression, grief, generalized anxiety, family problems, marital or sex issues, problems at work, desire for weight loss, drug and alcohol issues, and eating disorders. In other words, they appeared for therapy for the same reasons as those in the *Consumer Reports* study. In this same study, 97% ranked therapist competence as fair to excellent, and all of the participants were satisfied to completely satisfied with their therapist. Similarly, *Consumer Reports* respondents were equally pleased whether they were seen by a psychiatrist, psychologist, or social worker. According to the investigator, "These similarities suggest that the experience of persons who receive mental health services may transcend many significant differences, such as type of therapy, method, severity of diagnosis or cognitive ability" (p. 151).

Of particular importance are the quantitative improvement measures as a result of taking part in the IBT groups. Ninety percent of the participants felt that therapy improved their ability to get along with others, while 82.5% believed it helped them become more productive at work. Eighty percent felt it helped them cope with everyday stress, and 85% felt IBT helped them enjoy life more. In addition, 92.5% thought that therapy was responsible for personal growth and insight, while 95% noted that their confidence and self-esteem had been bettered. Concerning combating the symptoms of depression, the most commonly sought-after reason for treatment, 85% felt IBT helped them alleviate low moods. What is most striking about these numbers is that of the 40 participants, *none* reported that the therapy made them worse, even though this was a clear option they could have chosen (Lundrigan, 2007).

In-depth interviews offered additional insight as to what value the group process has for therapeutic gain. Although only carried out with five participants, the members reported they not only enjoyed receiving help from the group, but they also relished the opportunity to give it. This is emblematic of Yalom's original work (Yalon, 1995) on group psychotherapy and therapeutic factors, particularly when it is understood in the light of the therapeutic factors of altruism and guidance.

> In therapy groups, too, patients receive through giving, not only as part of the reciprocal giving-receiving sequence but also from the intrinsic act of giving. Psychiatric patients beginning therapy are demoralized and possess a deep sense of having nothing of value to offer others. They have long considered themselves as burdens, and the experience of finding that they can be of support to others is refreshing and boosts self-esteem (p. 12).

Although these studies are few in number with small sample sizes, they reflect the potentiality of the model and the need for more research. In general, until more research becomes available, clinicians will need to continue to adapt interventions from other populations.

The Virtual Gratitude Visit (VGV)

One of the original interventions developed for gratitude was by Martin Seligman who had students write letters of appreciation to people they felt had been kind but had not been thanked adequately (Seligman et al., 2005). For their gratitude visit, participants wrote and delivered letters of gratitude to these recipients. Compared to other interventions, those who performed the gratitude visit were found in the short-run to be the least depressed and the happiest of all the participants. The results from this intervention might be considered one of the early demonstrations of enhancing the character strength of gratitude directly. Additionally, gratitude has been found to enhance self-esteem (McCullough et al., 2002), life satisfaction (Kashdan et al., 2006), prosocial behavior (Wood et al., 2008), and better interpersonal relationships (Tsang, 2007). It was found to directly influence the capacity to broaden and build positive emotions (Fredrickson, 2004), and was noted as one of the primary interventions that can lead to sustainable happiness (Lyubomirsky et al., 2005). Importantly, it seems to also be a protective factor with depression (Ohlan & Gera, 2022). Gratitude, as has been said, may be the queen of virtues (Emmons, 2012).

For people with IDD who cannot read or write, crafting a gratitude letter and delivering it creates a barrier. The virtual gratitude visit was devised to eliminate limitations in expressing the strength-based emotion of gratitude. It uses role-playing with an empty chair and role reversal to enact an imaginary visit. It was originally designed to be used within the P-IBT format during the enactment stage.

The VGV builds on the research focused on the enhanced power of expressing gratitude to others in ways other than writing. Prior research compared a gratitude journal group to a similar group that also verbally expressed their gratitude. The researchers found that the expressive group did better than gratitude journaling alone or the control group. In the expressing-to-others group, negative emotions and depression decreased, which provided greater emotional balance. The authors concluded that other-oriented gratitude is enhanced when it is outwardly expressed. This research moves away from written expression to a powerful form of verbal expression (Goldstein & Winner, 2012). To extrapolate, the VGV employs this essence of verbal expression to others by using an empty chair by way of a psychodramatic role-play. The technique builds on the work in drama therapy (Tomasulo & Szucs, 2016), psychodrama (Fong, 2006), and role-playing (Nikzadeh & Soudani, 2016), each of which describe enactment methods shown to offer therapeutic gains (Kipper & Ritchie, 2003).

Within the structure of a P-IBT format, the orientation and warm-up and sharing stages are designed to prepare the group for interaction and participation. During the enactment stage, elements of role-playing are introduced as a way to capture the attention and interest of the participants and capitalize on the previous stage's preparation. In using the virtual gratitude visit, the orientation and warm-up and sharing is geared toward a conversation about people who have been kind to oneself and the appreciation for them. In the orientation stage, listening to and feeding back to people what they heard about the people they have gratitude for helps create the theme and activates the therapeutic factor of universality. As a result, when the group moves to warm-up and sharing, there is greater cohesion. Therapeutic factors (e.g., cohesion and universality) along with character strengths (e.g., love and kindness) are expressed and acknowledged by the facilitator(s).

During the enactment stage, the VGV is set up typically by having a protagonist volunteer to come into the center of the group and sit across from an empty chair (if they are willing). As the VGV uses role-playing with an empty chair to enact a gratitude visit, the intervention can include unavailable others. This significantly broadens the applicability of the technique. The person can be present in their life now, passed several years ago, or someone they have lost touch with. Importantly the person has been selected because they have delivered kindness to the protagonist, and they may not have been adequately thanked.

For this technique, two chairs are arranged, one for the protagonist and the second the (auxiliary) empty chair for the other. The protagonist arranges the chairs in a way that symbolically depicts the relationship; that is, are the chairs close? Far apart? Side by side? One behind the other? The chairs' arrangement sets the emotional tone for the role play. The protagonist then sits in his or her chair and expresses gratitude toward the imagined other in the empty chair. Following this, the protagonist *reverses roles* and becomes the auxiliary. In doing so, the protagonist responds as if the gratitude had just been expressed to him or her. This auxiliary role is then relinquished, and the protagonist returns to the original chair, saying a closing remark or gesture to bring the scene to a close. This ends the enactment. While space limitations do not allow for a detailed discussion on the power of a role reversal in this technique, the understanding accrued by reversing to the other role employs elements of empathy and learning of the other through the theory of mind (Goldsteing & Winner, 2012). This role reversal also allows for an amplification of the positivity of gratitude and integration as it is experienced as both sender and receiver.

The protagonist starts and ends in their chair, expresses gratitude, reverses roles, and then returns. This allows for an optimal amount of integration. Following this, the group is invited to comment on what they witnessed. These comments are reflections about who their person might be and also how they felt as the protagonist went through the role-play. Typically, this is a time that deepens cohesion and universality. It also typically inspires hope and is a display of the therapeutic factor of modeling.

VGV is but one example of using evidence-informed interventions in newly configured ways. Practitioners should continue this effort in extrapolating from the myriad of character strengths interventions and select those they believe will engender the greatest benefit. By making adaptations to fit the various cognitive, adaptive, and cultural needs of those being served, we can extend the promising applications of character strengths to people with IDD.

Future Directions

There are three primary areas for future development with respect to advancement for treatment for people with the dual diagnosis of intellectual and psychiatric disabilities. The first is about accessibility to the VIA Survey and interventions using character strengths in order to more directly embed character strengths into treatment plans. This may involve reconceptualization of how the tool is administered to people with low or no literacy or poor attention spans. Second, it is critical that effort is made to include individuals with dual-diagnosis into research protocols involving positive interventions, positive psychotherapy, and strength-based treatment and programing. Finally, more extensive use of evidence-based interventions validated on neurotypical populations, modified to become evidence-informed interventions for these individuals, is needed. This would allow for a more rapid deployment of known effective interventions operating with needed modifications.

Key Takeaways

- Dual diagnosis (DD) is the coexistence of intellectual/developmental disability (IDD) and at least one psychiatric disorder. The mental health needs of people with IDD is more than three times higher than the general population.
- Treatment by society of people with IDD shifted from optimism, to the protection of the individual, to the protection of society. This has been a setback in developing psychological, educational, and behavioral technology.
- The Willowbrook Consent Decree was a major contributing factor to the passage of the Civil Rights of Institutionalized Persons Act of 1980. This legal turning point in treatment and care for individuals with IDD was ushered in through a psychological emphasis on behavioral management and applying behavioral principles. Despite these efforts, the field since 1980 has been dominated by ameliorating deficit behaviors, not cultivating strengths.
- There are a number of challenges in conducting research that includes people with IDD. Researchers and practitioners must continue to find ways to address the limitations while searching for coexisting strengths by developing measurement tools and cultivating character.
- Introducing and discussing VIA character strengths can likely build self-knowledge, self-understanding, and self-esteem for individuals with intellectual and/or developmental disabilities and those with a dual-diagnosis.
- The *Diagnostic Manual for People with IDD* (DM-ID 2) is an evidence-based manual highlighting the shift in diagnostic criteria used for people with IDD and particularly useful for dual-diagnosis.
- Interactive-Behavioral Therapy (IBT) and later Positive-Interactive Behavioral therapy (P-IBT) are forms of group psychotherapy that have been shown to be effective with people with IDD.
- P-IBT facilitators affirm features that sanction and facilitate therapeutic elements of group dynamics while reinforcing the expression of individual character strengths.
- For people with IDD who cannot read or write, crafting a gratitude letter and delivering it creates a barrier. The virtual gratitude visit was devised to eliminate limitations in the expression of the character strength of gratitude. It uses role-playing with an empty chair and role-reversal to enact an imaginary visit. This character strengths intervention can include those who are unavailable, significantly broadening access to the feeling.

References

Albaum, C., Chan, V., Sellitto, T., Vashi, N., Hastings, R. P., & Weiss, J. A. (2021). Redressing the balance: A systematic review of positive psychology in the IDD literature. *International Review of Research in Developmental Disabilities, 60*, 1–53.

Aman, M. G., & Handen, B. (2006). Reactions to "Ethical challenges and complexities of including people with IDD as participants in research" by Dr Teresa Iacono. *Journal of Intellectual and Developmental Disability, 31*(3), 180–182.

American Psychiatric Association. (2000). *Diagnostic and statistical manual of mental disorders.* 4th edn. *Text Revision* (*DSM-IV-TR*). American Psychiatric Association.

American Psychological Association, APA Task Force on Guidelines for Assessment and Intervention with Persons with Disabilities. (2022). *Guidelines for assessment and intervention with persons with disabilities*. Retrieved from https://www.apa.org/about/policy/guidelines-assessment-intervention-disabilities.pdf

Beadle-Brown, J., Beecham, J., Leigh, J., Whelton, R., & Richardson, L. (2021). Outcomes and costs of skilled support for people with severe or profound IDD and complex needs. *Journal of Applied Research in IDD, 34*(1), 42–54.

Blaine, C. (1993). *Interpersonal learning in short-term integrated group psychotherapy* (Unpublished Master's thesis). University of Alberta.

Brown, I., Brown, R. I., Edwards, M., Bertelli, M. O., & Schalock, R. L. (2022). Quality of life as an outcome measure. In M. O. Bertelli, S. Deb, K. Munir, A. Hassiotis, & L. Salvador-Carulla (Eds.), *Textbook of psychiatry for IDD and autism spectrum disorder* (pp. 349–367). Springer.

Buckley, N., Glasson, E. J., Chen, W., Epstein, A., Leonard, H., Skoss, R., et al. (2020). Prevalence estimates of mental health problems in children and adolescents with IDD: A systematic review and meta-analysis. *Australian & New Zealand Journal of Psychiatry, 54*(10), 970–984.

Carlin, M. (1998). *Death, bereavement, and grieving: A group intervention for bereaved individuals with cerebral palsy* (Unpublished doctoral dissertation). C.W. Post Campus, Long Island University, USA.

Charlson, F., van Ommeren, M., Flaxman, A., Cornett, J., Whiteford, H., & Saxena, S. (2019). New WHO prevalence estimates of mental disorders in conflict settings: A systematic review and meta-analysis. *The Lancet, 394*(10194), 240–248.

Daniels, L. (1998). A group cognitive–behavioral and process-oriented approach to treating the social impairment and negative symptoms associated with chronic mental illness. *Journal of Psychotherapy Research and Practice, 7*, 167–176.

Dattani, S., Ritchie, H., & Roser, M. (2021). *Mental health*. Published online at OurWorldInData.org. Retrieved from: https://ourworldindata.org/mental-health [Online Resource].

Dean, E. E., Shogren, K. A., Hagiwara, M., & Wehmeyer, M. L. (2018). How does employment influence health outcomes? A systematic review of the IDD literature. *Journal of Vocational Rehabilitation, 49*(1), 1–13.

Emmons, R. A. (2012). Queen of the virtues? Gratitude as human strength. *Reflective Practice: Formation and Supervision in Ministry, 32*.

Fletcher, R. J., Barnhill, J., & Cooper, S.-A. (2017). *DM-ID 2. Diagnostic manual—IDD: A textbook of diagnosis of mental dis- orders in persons with IDD*. NADD- National Association for the Dually Diagnosed.

Flückiger, C., & Grosse Holtforth, M. (2008). Focusing the therapist's attention on the patient's strengths: A preliminary study to foster a mechanism of change in outpatient psychotherapy. *Journal of Clinical Psychology, 64*(7), 876–890.

Fong, J. (2006). Psychodrama as a preventive measure: Teenage girls confronting violence. *Journal of Group Psychotherapy, Psychodrama & Sociometry, 59*(3), 99–108.

Fredrickson, B. L. (2004). Gratitude, like other positive emotions, broadens and builds. In R. A. Emmons & M. E. McCullough (Eds.), *The psychology of gratitude* (pp. 145–166). Oxford University Press.

Giacomucci, S. (2021). Psychodrama practice in clinical social work with individuals. In *Social work, sociometry, and psychodrama* (pp. 323–342). Springer.

Goldstein, T. R., & Winner, E. (2012). Enhancing empathy and theory of mind. *Journal of Cognition and Development, 13*(1), 19–37.

Guercio, J. M. (2020). The importance of a deeper knowledge of the history and theoretical foundations of behaviorism and behavior therapy: Part 2—1960–1985. *Behavior Analysis: Research and Practice, 20*(3), 174–195. https://doi.org/10.1037/bar0000178

Harzer, C., & Ruch, W. (2015). The relationships of character strengths with coping, work- related stress, and job satisfaction. *Frontiers in Psychology, 6*(165), 1–12. https://doi.org/10.3389/fpsyg.2015.00165

Herat, M. (2021). Historical learning disabilities: Linguistic abilities of ex-servicemen with 'imbecility', 'feeblemindedness' and 'mental deficiency' in the ministry of pension files. In *Epistolary constructions of Post-World War I identity* (pp. 65–90). Palgrave.

Iacono, T. (2006). Ethical challenges and complexities of including people with IDD as participants in research. *Journal of Intellectual and Developmental Disability, 31*(3), 173–179.

Ilyes, E. (2020). Psychology's eugenic history and the invention of IDD. *Social and Personality Psychology Compass, 14*(7), e12537.

Kashdan, T. B., Uswatte, G., & Julian, T. (2006). Gratitude and hedonic and eudaimonic well-being in Vietnam war veterans. *Behaviour Research and Therapy, 44*, 177–199.

Keller E (1995). *Process and outcomes in interactive-behavioral groups with adults who have both mental illness and mental retardation* (Unpublished doctoral dissertation). C.W. Post Campus, Long Island University, USA.

Kipper, D. A., & Ritchie, T. D. (2003). The effectiveness of psychodramatic techniques: A meta-analysis. *Group Dynamics: Theory Research and Practice, 7*(1), 13–25.

Littman-Ovadia, H., Lazar-Butbul, V., & Benjamin, B. A. (2014). Strengths-based career counseling: Overview and initial evaluation. *Journal of Career Assessment, 22*(3), 403–419. https://doi.org/10.1177/1069072713498483

Luckasson, R., Tassé, M. J., & Schalock, R. L. (2022). Professional responsibility in the field of intellectual and developmental disabilities: Its definition, application, and impacts. *Intellectual and Developmental Disabilities, 60*(3), 183–198.

Lundrigan, M. (2007). *Interactive behavioral therapy with intellectually disabled persons with psychiatric disorders: A pragmatic case study*. (Psy.D Thesis). Graduate School of Applied and Professional Psychology, Rutgers University, USA.

Lysaght, R., Ouellette-Kuntz, H., & Lin, C. J. (2012). Untapped potential: Perspectives on the employment of people with IDD. *Work, 41*(4), 409–422.

Lyubomirsky, S., Sheldon, K. M., & Schkade, D. (2005). Pursuing happiness: The architecture of sustainable change. *Review of General Psychology, 9*, 111–131.

Maulik, P. K., Mascarenhas, M. N., Mathers, C. D., Dua, T., & Saxena, S. (2011). Prevalence of IDD: a meta-analysis of population-based studies. *Research in Developmental Disabilities, 32*(2), 419–436.

Mazza, M. G., Rossetti, A., Crespi, G., & Clerici, M. (2020). Prevalence of co-occurring psychiatric disorders in adults and adolescents with IDD: A systematic review and meta-analysis. *Journal of Applied Research in IDD, 33*(2), 126–138.

McConkey, R., Craig, S., & Kelly, C. (2019). The prevalence of IDD: A comparison of national census and register records. *Research in Developmental Disabilities, 89*, 69–75.

McCullough, M. E., Emmons, R., & Tsang, J. (2002). The grateful disposition: A conceptual and empirical topography. *Journal of Personality and Social Psychology, 82*, 112–127.

Niemiec, R. M., Shogren, K. A., & Wehmeyer, M. L. (2017). Character strengths and intellectual and developmental disability: A strengths-based approach from positive psychology. *Education and Training in Autism and Developmental Disabilities, 52*(1).

Nikzadeh, E., & Soudani, M. (2016). *Evaluating the effectiveness of drama therapy by psychodrama method on psychological wellbeing and false beliefs of addicts* (pp. 148–155). Canadian Center of Science and Education.

Ohlan, A., & Gera, T. (2022). Character strength of hope and gratitude as protective factor of suicide. *Journal of Positive School Psychology, 6*(9), 2732–2739.

Oliver-Brannon, G. (2000). *Counseling and psychotherapy in group treatment with the dually diagnosed (mental retardation and mental illness—MR/MI)* (Doctoral dissertation). The Union Institute, 2000. Dissertation Abstracts International 60(10–B): 5230.

Peterson, C., & Seligman, M. E. (2004). *Character strengths and virtues: A handbook and classification*. Oxford University Press and American Psychological Association.

Raley, S. K., Shogren, K. A., & Cole, B. P. (2020). Positive psychology and education of students with disabilities: The way forward for assessment and intervention. *Advances in Neurodevelopmental Disorders, 5*, 11. https://doi.org/10.1007/s41252-020-00181-8

Rashid, T. (2020). Positive psychotherapy. In *Encyclopedia of quality of life and well-being research* (pp. 1–8). Springer International Publishing.

Rashid, T., & Seligman, M. P. (2018). *Positive psychotherapy: Clinician manual*. Oxford University Press.

Razza, N. J., & Tomasulo, D. J. (2005). *Healing trauma: The power of group treatment for people with IDD*. American Psychological Association.

Reinders, J., Stainton, T., & Parmenter, T. R. (2019). The quiet progress of the new eugenics. Ending the lives of persons with intellectual and developmental disabilities for reasons of presumed poor quality of life. *Journal of Policy and Practice in IDD, 16*(2), 99–112.

Reiss, S., Levitan, G. W., & Szyszko, J. (1982). Emotional disturbance and mental retardation: diagnostic overshadowing. *American Journal of Mental Deficiency, 86*, 567–574.

Schalock, R. L., Luckasson, R., & Tassé, M. J. (2021). An overview of IDD: Definition, diagnosis, classification, and systems of supports. *American Journal on Intellectual and Developmental Disabilities, 126*(6), 439–442.

Schwartz, A. E., Caoili, A., Beasley, J. B., Kramer, J. M., & Kalb, L. G. (2022). Clinical applications of the VIA inventory of strengths with individuals with intellectual/developmental disabilities. *Journal of Positive Psychology*. https://doi.org/10.1080/17439760.2022.2036797

Scior, K., Hamid, A., Hastings, R., Werner, S., Belton, C., Laniyan, A., et al. (2020). IDD stigma and initiatives to challenge it and promote inclusion around the globe. *Journal of Policy and Practice in IDD, 17*(2), 165–175.

Seligman, M. E. P. (1995). The effectiveness of psychotherapy: The consumer reports study. *American Psychologist, 50*(12), 965–974.

Seligman, M. E. P. (2002). Positive psychology, positive prevention, and positive therapy. *Handbook of Positive Psychology, 2*(2002), 3–12.

Seligman, M. E. P., Steen, T. A., Park, N., & Peterson, C. (2005). Positive psychology progress: Empirical validation of interventions. *American Psychologist, 60*(5), 410.

Shogren, K. A., Niemiec, R. M., Tomasulo, D., & Khamsi, S. (2017). Character strengths. In M. Wehmeyer (Ed.), *Handbook of positive psychology in intellectual and developmental disabilities* (pp. 189–199). Springer.

Shogren, K. A., Shaw, L. A., Raley, S. K., Wehmeyer, M. L., Niemiec, R. M., & Adkins, M. (2018). Assessing character strengths in youth with IDD: Reliability and factorial validity of the VIA-youth. *Intellectual and Developmental Disabilities, 56*(1), 13–29.

Singh, N. N., Lancioni, G. E., Winton, A. S. W., Singh, A. N., Adkins, A. D., & Singh, J. (2009). Mindful staff can reduce the use of physical restraints when providing care to individuals with IDD. *Journal of Applied Research in IDD, 22*, 194–202. https://doi.org/10.1111/j.1468-3148.2008.00488.x

Tomasulo, D. J. (2014). Positive group psychotherapy modified for adults with IDD. *Journal of IDD, 18*(4), 337–350.

Tomasulo, D. (2018). American snake pit: Hope, grit, and resilience in the wake of Willowbrook. .

Tomasulo, D., & Szucs, A. (2016). The ACTing cure: Evidence-based group treatment for people with IDD. *Dramatherapy., 37*, 100. https://doi.org/10.1080/02630672.2016.1162824

Tsang, J. (2007). Gratitude for small and large favors: A behavioral test. *The Journal of Positive Psychology, 2*, 157–167.

UN General Assembly. (2006). *Convention on the rights of persons with disabilities*, A/RES/61/106, Annex I, available at: https://www.refwo rld.org/docid/4680cd212.html. Accessed 15 Nov 2022.

Vereenooghe, L., Flynn, S., Hastings, R. P., Adams, D., Chauhan, U., Cooper, S. A., et al. (2018). Interventions for mental health problems in children and adults with severe IDD: a systematic review. *BMJ Open, 8*(6), e021911.

Werner, S., & Stawski, M. (2012). Mental health: knowledge, attitudes and training of professionals on dual diagnosis of IDD and psychiatric disorder. *Journal of IDD Research, 56*(3), 291–304.

Wood, A. M., Joseph, S., & Maltby, J. (2008). Gratitude uniquely predicts satisfaction with life: Incremental validity above the domains and facets of the five factor model. *Personality and Individual Differences, 45*, 49–54.

Yalom, I. (1995). *The theory and practice of group psychotherapy* (4th ed.). Basic Books.

Yin, L. C., & Majid, R. A. (2018). The goodness of character strengths in education. *International Journal of Academic Research in Business and Social Sciences, 8*(6), 1237–1251.

Chapter 9
Justice, Equity, Diversity, and Inclusion (JEDI) and Intellectual/Developmental Disabilities

The only thing necessary for the triumph of evil is for good men to do nothing.

-Often attributed to Edmund Burke

The Concepts

Positive psychology has been criticized for its lack of inclusion for various underrepresented groups. Issues of gender, race, and ethnicity have been unevenly balanced and there has been a frequent reliance on WEIRD (Western, Educated, Industrialized, Rich, Democratic) samples, although this has been improving in the last decade with increasing globalization of positive psychology and increasing representation from non-Western countries (Hendriks et al., 2019). As an example, women are traditionally overrepresented as participants in research but underrepresented as first authors. Research subjects in published studies are frequently Caucasian, literate, and do not include research on the intersection of such factors as gender, race and ethnicity (Rao & Donaldson, 2015).

Suggestions have been made for improvement in the areas of research design, authorship, research topics, and greater inclusion of information on gender, race and ethnicity. It would be fair to say that the need and these suggestions are frequently being welcomed in many contexts, but at the same time they only represent the beginning of broadening the scope and impact of research in positive psychology.

More specifically, the research on character strengths may represent one aspect of positive psychology where the conditions and foundation for insight into justice, equity, diversity, and inclusion may be more fertile and amenable to advances. This is because the construction of the VIA Classification of character strengths (Peterson & Seligman, 2004) began with a desire to understand the universal human experience, that is, what is best and common across cultures, nations, and beliefs. In other words, the classification began by trying to look at human virtues and strengths not

R. M. Niemiec, D. Tomasulo, *Character Strengths and Abilities Within Disabilities*, Positive Psychology and Disability Series,
https://doi.org/10.1007/978-3-031-36294-1_9

limited to a particular group. As such the VIA Survey provides a means for comparison while drawing from principles extracted from universal principles, thus embracing the whole of humanity and tailoring it to the individual. To further this point, the translation of the VIA Survey or VIA Youth Survey has been done (and validated) in more than 50 languages. This more universal approach has, by definition, justice, equity, diversity, and inclusion (JEDI) woven (to some degree) into the tapestry of this work. Character strengths may reflect a platform that allows for the deepening of our understanding and expansion of each of these concerns.

While it would be beyond the scope of this chapter to highlight the vast scope implied by issues of JEDI, as well as the many movements, missions, historical and contemporary work in these areas, a more tailored approach is offered.

This chapter will focus on character strengths as they relate to justice, equity, diversity, and inclusion for people with intellectual/developmental disability (IDD). Arguably, this highly underserved population represents the difficulties and potentiality behind the use of character strengths in practice. People with IDD may be emblematic as a group that is typically ignored, stigmatized, minimalized, and yet greatly in need of services. We have chosen this group in particular because they frequently lack a voice, the ability to demand resources, point out their inequities, or protest their treatment, although this is changing by the movement of self-advocates as well as supportive groups helping to enable self-advocacy and change. They represent what our profession needs to be doing to meet the needs of others separate from what a group might do to bring attention to their needs. Serving the needs of justice and equity cannot rely solely on the voice of activists. Diversity and inclusion need to be principle-derived through the intent of the researcher and practitioner. While this is meant to offer an example of how character strengths are being applied to this population in relationship to JEDI, the hope is it may also serve as a template for appreciating the challenges and opportunities of applying character strengths to an underrepresented population.

There is an interconnection among the four areas of JEDI in that to talk about one is to talk about the other three, to some degree. We offer some distinctions, however, one must keep that wider reality in mind. In addition, it is the character strengths that can offer unique pathways enabling, facilitating, and even embodying justice, equity, diversity, and inclusion.

The Science

JEDI and Character Strengths

Nearly 1 billion people in the world cannot read this sentence. Yet, most positive psychology interventions involve the ability to read and write. In particular, the main tool in the field of positive psychology, the VIA Survey, is not available in an alternate form for individuals with no literacy at the time of this writing. While the use of a third party can support individuals without literacy, greater accessibility to the individuals themselves would allow for a better understanding of signature strengths, better understanding of the collective strengths of people with IDD, and their comparison to other disabilities.

The value of the VIA Survey for the development of strength-based interventions to foster self-esteem, self-understanding, and self-knowledge, as well as to provide cross-system service coordination has been highlighted (Schwartz et al., 2022). Having a strengths-based platform to promote the infusion of character strengths into daily programs for people with IDD would extend the reach of the VIA Survey to individuals who may need it the most (Niemiec et al., 2017).

Such availability would offer the VIA to a greater diversity of individuals with direct access. This would grant people with IDD a more direct right of entry to the character strengths work as other marginalized groups. This information not only adds to strengthen the utility of a strength-based approach for people with IDD, it broadens the extent to which a more diverse population of users can be directly measured (Umucu, et al., 2022).

Equity and Character Strengths

When equity is applied to individuals with IDD, there is a thin line easily crossed when it comes to the practices of fairness. This line is between equity and marginalization. If we scaffold treatments, education, and services to make them more accessible and applicable to people with IDD, it may be ostracizing and alienating the very individual we are hoping to help (Shifrer et al., 2013).

The issues that fuel the need for equity are most often rooted in associations outside conscious awareness. Often this bias is based on irrelevant, inaccurate, or imagined perspective that leads to a negative, dismissive, or marginalized evaluation of a person.

From emergency room treatment to psychotherapy health care, providers routinely marginalize people with IDD. Under the umbrella of diagnostic overshadowing (discussed in Chaps. 5 and 8), triage for treatment, and inadequate training, professionals may not offer services. If they do, it will often be inadequate and indicative of an implicit bias (FitzGerald & Hurst, 2017). This type of bias creates disparities influencing diagnosis, treatment decisions, and level of care.

Education of professionals about implicit bias allows for a deliberate approach toward ameliorating the problem. Accepting people where they are, however, is an ongoing, evolving project, and building education into training curriculum, offering continuing education credits, and fostering research may be good ways to increase awareness concerning the problem of these biases.

But education alone is not the answer. A more robust intervention is to offer alternatives to implicit bias that directly counteract the perspective. Toward this end a description of a pilot study may help to explain the approach. Emergency room physicians have a tough job because they are constantly evaluating and balancing the resources and needs of incoming patients. Quick decisions that rely on years of training and education come to the front of mind in a matter of seconds.

People with IDD, have greater and more complex needs when admitted to an emergency room, and are often not prioritized. This has been hypothesized to be at least partially due to an implicit bias and diagnostic overshadowing. While awareness and education of this issue is certainly important, another approach in its developmental stages may be an important consideration.

If an implicit bias is at work during the diagnosis and treatment, adding another evaluative tool can be helpful. For example, emergency room physicians could be taught about character strengths and how they are universal and after the training taught about strength-spotting. People with IDD when entering an emergency room accompanied by a staff person can let the staff know of the patient's signature strengths. In addition to the medical history and evaluation, character strengths are discussed to begin counteracting a potential implicit bias. Those not accompanied by staff could be assessed through strength-spotting and asking questions such as, "What do you like to do when you are not visiting us?" The answers can reveal a few of the individual's top strengths, which can then be capitalized on by staff and physicians. This type of approach also enhances the perspective of those with less bias, while helping to balance the perspective of those who have more substantial biases. While potentially helping to correct an implicit bias and increase patient morale, it facilitates human-to-human interactions during a difficult time. It allows for mainstream care without marginalization.

Inclusion and Character Strengths

The official principles behind such initiatives like the mental health act and the human rights act advocate the right of people with intellectual disability to lead their lives with dignity and respect. Additionally, what is explicitly endorsed is that they should have the same opportunities and responsibilities afforded to them as anyone else (Hollins et al., 2019).

However, in two major areas, education and mental health, these initiatives are often met with a disparity between the needs and resources of the facilities and individuals providing education or treatment. It is well known that people with IDD are more susceptible to mental health issues and needs than the general population (Buckles et al., 2013). The cognitive deficits that are concomitant with an intellectual disability often provide obstacles on the path to learning. Psychological issues that may need modified treatment protocols or the capacity for insight to be effective may also be challenges to mental health professionals working with people with IDD. This makes access to effective mental health services problematic at both systemic and personal levels (Whittle et al., 2019).

Yet, in spite of these hurdles noncognitive qualities, such as reflected in character strengths, may provide the most effective and dynamic approach to education and well-being.

In education, people with intellectual disabilities are frequently separated from main classes to resource rooms for specialized instruction. Following this or concomitantly they are integrated into mainstream classrooms, often with the support of an aid. Yet the vast majority of these programs rely on skill-based and intellectual properties. They look to deficits in these two areas and seek to improve and enhance disabilities.

But in the field of education there has been a radical shift to support character education alongside traditional curriculum. This means awareness of and application of character development is brought alongside traditional education. The results of this approach have been well documented and show gains in better grade point averages, lower conduct disorders, less depression, and higher well-being. Students who develop their character do better in school (Seligman & Adler, 2018).

In the field of mental health, it has been a long-standing problem that people with intellectual disabilities have been perceived as inappropriate, unresponsive, or unable to profit from treatment. This has not been true, although the implicit bias of professionals is a true and strong influence. Recent advances in mental health treatment for people with intellectual disabilities suggests that what has happened in the field of education may be possible in the psychological treatment of people with IDD. By focusing on character development as part of a treatment plan, people with IDD may benefit in terms of self-esteem, self-knowledge, and self-efficacy.

The VIA Survey involved a more comprehensive and holistic approach in its development than most other instruments in psychology. The VIA Institute, which houses the VIA Survey and VIA Classification, maintains a World Database on Character, with billions of data-points and 30-million VIA Survey takers (at the time of this writing. It provides access to measures and database queries to anyone in the world looking to research the patterns or utility of character strengths. Because of this large accessability there is a foundation for Justice, Equity, Diversity, and Inclusion to have a common portal, and studies in this vein are in process. This platform may offer insights into how best to identify needs before they become tragic consequences and implement needed changes.

Research on JEDI and Intellectual/Developmental Disabilities begins with the understanding that other non-IDD marginalized groups have two major advantages. First, they have the intellectual and organizing ability to self-advocate for their needs. Second, they have the capacity to use their academic influence to show evidence-based rationale for their concerns. More global concerns such as gender, race, and ethnicity as they relate to JEDI are examples of how such under-represented groups are capable of promoting their positions (Rao & Donaldson, 2015).

For context on justice for people with IDD the reader is directed to a seminal work on the societal, legal, social, and political implications of the Willowbrook Decree and its influence on the Civil Rights of Institutionalized Persons Act of 1980. Revealed in *The Willowbrook Wars: Bringing the Mentally Disabled into the Community* (Rothman, 2017) are details of the story and legal battle that changed mental health services in America. Additionally, a more personal account can be found in *American Snake Pit: Hope, Grit, and Resilience in the Wake of Willowbrook* (Tomasulo, 2018).

Character strengths development is tethered specifically to the need for justice for people with intellectual disability by directly addressing the need for human dignity. Yet, more than addressing the character strengths of people with IDD, it is the character strengths activation of people awakened by the need for dignity in others (Sheldon & Schüler, 2011) that is important to note when looking at the need for justice. As many people with IDD cannot self-advocate, their plight must be recognized and appreciated by those who can advocate on their behalf or support them. The vehicle for this, whether it be in the courtroom, newspaper, book, or movie, is storytelling. The story can be told through a news video that changes the political climate (Valldejuli, 2022), or through a memoir (Tomasulo, 2018), or through courtroom narrative (Dvoskin et al., 2020). It is the basis of storytelling that helps for purpose and meaning to be crystallized (Smith, 2017). These stories—how, where, and to whom they are told—become the basis for either systemic changes (Whittle et al., 2019) or personal changes (FitzGerald & Hurst, 2017).

Within the area of inclusion there has been compelling arguments and rationale for the infusion of character strengths into the advancement of mental health systems for IDD (Niemiec et al., 2017). There is emerging literature that the character development woven into traditional and modified protocols and psychotherapy has been successful. In the early years following the advent of the VIA Classification, character strengths were being suggested as an important part of a school counselor's approach by Peterson (Park & Peterson, 2008) and Seligman (Kobau et al., 2011). Since that time there has been a steady growth of literature focusing on strengths, optimal functioning, and the well-being of individuals with intellectual disabilities in therapeutic settings (Albaum et al., 2021). While keeping the focus on mental health treatment, there is good evidence and rationale to begin the recognition and focus on character strength-based practices in special education settings (Raley et al., 2021). This emphasis on the positive effect of character strengths awareness can begin early in schools and continue the life-long process of character development to achieve greater life satisfaction.

Although still early in development, the therapeutic community is finding strength-based treatment and training useful (Schwartz et al., 2022). It has clear rationale and evidence for not only continuing its use in general applications (Shogren et al., 2017a, b), but also alongside adaptation of specific methods like Dialectical Behavior Therapy (Seavey, 2012), group video feedback (Szucs et al., 2019), cinematherapy (Smieszek, 2019), mindfulness (Szucs et al., 2020), dramatherapy (Tomasulo & Szucs, 2015), and group psychotherapy (Tomasulo, 2015). In addition, with significant findings in recovery (Slade, 2010) and with acute psychiatric disabilities (Kouvaras et al., 2022), positive psychotherapy provides a manualized framework to impact multiple populations (Rashid, 2015, 2020; Rashid & Seligman, 2018).

Central to the success of IDD and JEDI applications is the initial foundation of awareness, understanding, and use of character strengths. This orientation features a highlighting of those positive features of oneself that can be cultivated through recognition and application of signature strengths. In the application of psychotherapy for people with intellectual disabilities, the addition of character strengths and emphasis on positivity and strengths represents a major shift in applying historically attempted therapeutic treatment for people with IDD (O'Driscoll, 2008; Thompson Prout & Browning, 2011) and their caregivers (Manesh, 2017).

The Practice

In spite of all the work being done by the science of psychology, including theory, methods, and research, true change and impact on treatment of individuals happens not as a result of science and research outcomes, but by a change in the laws that guide us. In some ways, policy change is the core practice needed.

This has been true in education (Klarman, 2007), affirmative action (Graham, 1992), and a patient's medical bill of rights (Annas, 2004), to name a few. Within the field of mental health, the same is also true. Mental health as a civil right in the United States grew out of the mistreatment of intellectually disabled individuals in a facility in Staten Island, New York, known as the Willowbrook State School. Before Willowbrook, the right to treatment for mental health while in an institution was not a concern. People could be treated as poorly or as well as the authorities would allow—and protection for the most vulnerable among us was not a consideration. It stands at the very nexus of JEDI issues in mental health and became the tipping point for mental health treatment and quality in the United States. It was only after decades of abuse and maltreatment that the conditions finally brought about a legal battle to make a change. In the end it would take more than 20 years, and over 100 court hearings to bring lasting differences. The system changed not because of good psychological intervention but because of powerful lawsuits that held people accountable for their action. This ushered in the opportunity for psychological science to facilitate the desired change.

The Willowbrook State School was a type of hell on earth, and in 1963, it had become[1] the largest state facility of its kind in the United States, forcing over 6000 residents into a space for 4275. Understaffed right from the beginning it was composed largely of medical personnel and refugee physicians from Hitler's Germany and Majority World (i.e., developing) countries. In 1964, a New York legislative committee toured the facility and was horrified at the abuse, neglect, and "vile stench." Their confidential report highlighted the cruelties and mismanagement, but it was not until the violent deaths, which all took place in the first half of 1965, that the institution made the news. A man and, later, a 10-year-old boy were scalded to death by a shower as a result of poor plumbing and unsophisticated attendants. One resident died from a punch in the throat by another inmate, and a 12-year-old strangled himself struggling to get free from a restraining device. These deaths and the resulting concerns made it into the local paper. It is often the case that it takes

[1]The information on Willowbrook is summarized and drawn from the author's (DT) memoir *American Snake Pit.*

catastrophes for enough attention to be paid to an issue and eventual mobilization of the legal system. Following these horrific events, Robert Kennedy, the then US senator from New York, showed up unannounced. He saw firsthand the conditions and told the press, "I think that particularly at Willowbrook, we have a situation that borders on a snake pit… living in filth and dirt, their clothing in rags, in rooms less comfortable and cheerful than the cages in which we put animals in a zoo." Even with all the bad press and the political watchdogs the conditions actually got worse. For justice to occur there needs to be a critical mass of concern. The fact that people with IDD generally lack the cognitive ability to organize protests and lobby for their cause indicates that the injustice must touch others.

Character strengths play many roles in fostering justice. Individuals high on fairness, courage, teamwork, and love might very well be those who head the cause. In this way it is not the character strengths of the individuals being affected that motivates initial change. It is those who witness their struggle and respond.

This is a delicate pivot point because it involves the intersection and vision of the situation through the dual lens of psychology and law. To understand this is to see the need for justice through the eyes of those who need it, and those who can bring it about.

The physician's perspective combined with the administrative neglect created intolerable conditions that had become so routine they were the norm. Psychologist Phil Zimbardo (2011) has dubbed this pattern *The Lucifer Effect.* Willowbrook, according to Zimbardo's work, had followed a pattern where individuals in institutions become numb to their atrocities and, as Zimbardo argues, evil becomes an accepted practice. The essence of justice rests squarely on the character strength of fairness. But what if the fairness of the governing authority is underused or overused? We could predict prejudice, partisanship, and detachment. Indeed, all the things found at Willowbrook.

History reveals no shortage of examples: the Holocaust, the Mai Lai Massacre in Vietnam, mass suicides in Guyana by the People's Temple, the Branch Davidians in Texas, and the torture of Iraqi prisoners by US soldiers at Abu Ghraib. Each shows how inhumanity becomes *a slow and insidious process of becoming culture.* In the case of Willowbrook, the unbalanced perspective of authorities demanded the initial resolution be legal—but the longer-term correction is psychological. At Willowbrook, the legal system would ultimately say what was happening is wrong and needed to change. But it would be the science of psychology that would craft and research how these changes become possible. In broad terms the legal system redefined and reestablished the definition of fairness. From a psychological perspective this was accomplished through the application of treatment goals which had been abandoned.

The problems in psychology as a science for the treatment of suffering can be traced back to the application of the medical model to psychological well-being. This is what was happening at Willowbrook. The psychiatrists at Willowbrook did not know better than to label the inmates as incurables. Through a physician's lens at that time, people with IDD were not capable of improving and no resources should be spent on them. Simply put, they were not worth spending money, time, or resources on. In fact, during this period much of the funding was being diverted to the war effort in Vietnam.

This medical approach fostered an environment and a protocol that fueled abuse and neglect. The inmates did not matter because it was believed they could not be improved. This erroneous assumption came from the distorted perspective that since the physicians did not know how to help, the patients could not improve. Ignorance and a lack of creativity, and the absence of fairness created an environment of abusive tolerance. At that time a physician would triage patients. Since the entire population of Willowbrook was deemed hopeless, no goals for improvement, dignity, education, or well-being were ever established. As one historian put it, Willowbrook had become "a dumping ground receiving discards as in a draw poker game." No effort toward rehabilitation was made and the emphasis became the most minimal custodial care. Without a treatment goal for improvement the facility became a warehouse for people.

Two enlightened physicians, Drs. Michael Wilkins and William Bronston, began reporting the deplorable conditions to the director. It is likely they exercised the character strengths of fairness, bravery, teamwork, leadership, perseverance, honesty, and love.

After unsuccessfully attempting to influence the administration (fairness and courage), Wilkins and Bronston took their platform to the parents' association of Willowbrook, the Benevolent Society (teamwork and love) who began protest demonstrations, and by December 1971 the parents were protesting regularly. Wilkins was fired in January. Wilkins told a friend of his, a lawyer named Geraldo Rivera who was working for New York Channel 7 news, that he still had the keys to the buildings at Willowbrook and suggested Rivera video the atrocities. These videos highlighted the atrocities, maltreatment, and institutionalized abuse that had been going on. It mobilized the legal system and eventually the Willowbrook Consent Decree became a major contributing force to the passage of the Civil Rights of Institutionalized Persons Act of 1980. This was the point in US history when mental health became a civil right.

The tragic impressions informed Americans about how evil replaces indifference: The parents, the public, and the lawmakers were both disgusted and motivated. Their character strengths expressions made the difference.

Now, because of Willowbrook, mental health became a civil right, people in any institution, nursing home, prison, or hospital had rights for treatment. What would be learned from Willowbrook is that when people are given a chance to feel safe and the opportunity to learn they can thrive. Oddly enough these opportunities would cost only a percentage of what it was to leave people untreated in the deplorable conditions of a poorly run institution.

While behaviorism was the predominant means through which psychological interventions were applied, the treatment goals were striving for changes in character. Although character strengths and their relationship to virtues and goodness had not yet been categorized and operationalized, the transformation rested on the elevation of human dignity. Character strength development fosters human dignity by developing habits of virtue (Morales-Sánchez & Cabello-Medina, 2015). In this way the behavioral modification efforts of the 1970s and 1980s strengthened positive behavioral responses while reducing negative or unwanted ones. As we change our habits to those with greater personal and societal value, we are developing human dignity through applying our character strengths (Sheldon & Schüler, 2011).

Case Example

This case study involves the meeting of two individuals, a man and a woman 30 years his senior, in Willowbrook. These two inmates (let us call them Jake and Fran) were kept in separate wards in the facility during its bleakest time. In an interview with this couple more than 30 years after their meeting, one author (DT) had the opportunity to hear the details of their journey together.

They each remember not having enough food or adequate clothing within the institution. They spoke about how unsafe it was, not just at the residence, but due to selected staff who used physical punishment and verbal threats to keep residents in line. Both Jake and Fran expressed in their own way a sense of hopelessness as well as the hopelessness of the situation. Yet, they laughed as they recalled how they knew the routines of each other and plotted ways they could watch as their yet to be partner would be walking with their group and pass where the other would be waiting to spot a glimpse of each other. "I knew she'd be waiting for me to walk with the others on the way to kitchen duty," he'd say with a smile. In separate and together interviews they both spoke about Geraldo Rivera and the aftermath of the legal process. They were both aware that they would not be out if it had not been for the legal battles.

Both highlighted the justice of the story and knowing specifically about the Willowbrook Decree as the legal precedent that allowed them to finally leave "that hell hole." Although they had met in the institution on a few occasions and enjoyed each other's company, they had never consummated the relationship and were then part of an initial group of high functioning individuals who were moved out as part of the Decree. They were both received by an agency in New York City. They were placed in different residences in the community, but were able to see one another at larger agency functions and social events sponsored by the agency. Having spent a lifetime in an institution they were unskilled and naïve about the dynamics of cultivating an intimate relationship.

The agency was, at that time, in the process of developing a dating service for people with intellectual disabilities in New York City. This avant-garde approach to bringing equity and relationship building to this population was also amplified by the development of psychoeducational groups. In these "dating" groups, people learned the dynamics of dating, the differences between friendship, acquaintances and dates, as well as being educated on the protocol of being on a date with someone you like, and want to pursue—versus being on a date with someone you did not. The range of topics in the curriculum ran the gamut from how to flirt to how to help put a condom on your partner. They had both taken part in this program to help bring a sense of decency, properness, and normalcy to their lives. The Decree gave them the freedom to want what everyone else would want.

After successfully learning to date Jake and Fran became exclusive. Several years later, they got engaged and sought help from a marriage counselor about managing their expectations of each other, and the concerns they would have about moving in together. The agency they were referred to for counseling, and eventually the counselor they were assigned to, had never had an intellectually disabled couple who had stayed together, gotten engaged, and were seeking marriage counseling. It is fair to say that the agency became more diverse because of taking on Jake and Fran, and the couple counselor went to get specialized training to become more effective.

They moved into an apartment that was financially sponsored by the agency. However, the apartment itself was in a regular New York City residential building. Like everyone else in the building, they were responsible for their apartment, negotiating their lives with other people, and taking care of all the day-to-day responsibilities such as buying food, preparing it, and doing household chores that come with a life together. Over time they became part of the fabric of this housing community, their neighborhood, their synagogue, and the collective social life in NYC. When Fran passed on, neighbors brought food for Jake, collected money for flowers, and some showed at the wake. Jake and Fran had become the very definition of inclusion.

The arc of their story rests on a panoply of character strengths that can be highlighted and we offer a few examples. There fortuitous meeting in Willowbrook was generated by the character strengths of *love*. It is clear that their *creativity* involved scheming ways to see one another, their *humor* as they reflected and retrospectively appreciated these small actions, their sense of *fairness* in knowing they had been treated unfairly, and their *gratitude* for Geraldo Rivera and the Willowbrook Decree. They showed *bravery* and *perseverance* as evidenced in moving out of a place they had lived for the greater part of their lives. There was the enduring *love* and shared *kindness* with each other, as well as *love of learning* as they moved into their apartment as a married couple. *Social intelligence* and *teamwork* can be observed in the finding of ways to become central to their residential community and neighborhood. Indeed, the argument could be made that each of the 24 strengths, including *forgiveness* for each other's transgressions and *spirituality* through finding meaning in their relationship and their attendance at the synagogue, could be found in their story. While the VIA Classification and VIA Survey were not yet developed, the principles upon which it was built were already deeply inherent in the lives of Jake and Fran.

Future Directions

We would expect new perspectives of various underserved populations to evolve as researchers from more diverse, marginalized populations publish their findings. For those marginalized groups that may lack the capacity to have members of their community conduct research, we look to other researchers to include more diverse populations into their existing studies. While this is true for positive psychology in general, it will particularly enrich our understanding of character strengths and their development and further our collective humanity.

Key Points

- Character strengths offer a pathway that allows for the deepening of our understanding and expansion of justice, equity, diversity, and inclusion.
- People with IDD may be emblematic as a group that is typically ignored, stigmatized, minimalized, and yet greatly in need of services.
- Mental health as a civil right in the United States grew out of the mistreatment of intellectually disabled individuals in a facility in Staten Island, New York, known as the Willowbrook State School.
- Willowbrook, according to Zimbardo's work, had followed a pattern where individuals in institutions become numb to their atrocities and, as Zimbardo argues, evil becomes an accepted practice.
- The medical approach at Willowbrook fostered an environment and a protocol that fueled abuse and neglect. The Willowbrook Consent Decree became a major contributing force to the passage of the Civil Rights of Institutionalized Persons Act of 1980. This was the point in US history when mental health became a civil right. Now, because of Willowbrook, mental health became a civil right for people in any institution, nursing home, prison, or hospital and thus giving them rights for treatment.
- Character strength development fosters human dignity by developing habits of virtue.
- Noncognitive qualities, such as reflected in character strengths, provide an effective and dynamic pathway for education and well-being.
- By focusing on character development as part of a treatment plan, people with IDD are being set up for higher self-esteem, self-knowledge, and self-efficacy.
- Character strengths development is tethered specifically to the need for justice for people with intellectual disability by directly addressing the needs for human dignity.
- As many people with IDD cannot self-advocate, their plight must be recognized and appreciated by those who can advocate on their behalf and support them. One vehicle for this, whether it be in the courtroom, newspaper, book, or movie, is storytelling.
- To expand the work of character strengths, including the VIA Classification and VIA Survey to support justice, equity, diversity and inclusion, effort needs to be made to make the work available to people of all capacities, and to become a foundational approach in the development of treatment plans, programs, and support services for individuals, staff and family.

References

Albaum, C., Chan, V., Sellitto, T., Vashi, N., Hastings, R. P., & Weiss, J. A. (2021). Redressing the balance: A systematic review of positive psychology in the intellectual disability literature. *International Review of Research in Developmental Disabilities, 60*, 1–53.

Annas, G. J. (2004). *The rights of patients: The authoritative ACLU guide to the rights of patients* (Vol. 1). NYU Press.

Buckles, J., Luckasson, R., & Keefe, E. (2013). A systematic review of the prevalence of psychiatric disorders in adults with intellectual disability, 2003–2010. *Journal of Mental Health Research in Intellectual Disabilities, 6*(3), 181–207.

Dvoskin, J. A., Knoll, J. L., & Silva, M. (2020). A brief history of the criminalization of mental illness. *CNS Spectrums, 25*(5), 638–650.

FitzGerald, C., & Hurst, S. (2017). Implicit bias in healthcare professionals: A systematic review. *BMC Medical Ethics, 18*(1), 1–18.

Graham, H. D. (1992). The origins of affirmative action: Civil rights and the regulatory state. *The Annals of the American Academy of Political and Social Science, 523*(1), 50–62.

Hendriks, T., Warren, M. A., Schotanus-Dijkstra, M., Hassankhan, A., Graafsma, T., Bohlmeijer, E., & de Jong, J. (2019). How WEIRD are positive psychology interventions? A bibliometric analysis of randomized controlled trials on the science of well-being. *The Journal of Positive Psychology, 14*(4), 489–501. https://doi.org/10.1080/17439760.2018.1484941

Hollins, S., Lodge, K. M., & Lomax, P. (2019). The case for removing intellectual disability and autism from the mental health act. *The British Journal of Psychiatry, 215*(5), 633–635.

Klarman, M. J. (2007). *Brown v. Board of Education and the civil rights movement*. Oxford University Press.

Kobau, R., Seligman, M. E., Peterson, C., Diener, E., Zack, M. M., Chapman, D., & Thompson, W. (2011). Mental health promotion in public health: Perspectives and strategies from positive psychology. *American Journal of Public Health, 101*(8), e1–e9.

Kouvaras, S., Guiotto, M., Schrank, B., Slade, M., & Riches, S. (2022). Character strength–focused positive psychotherapy on acute psychiatric wards: A feasibility and acceptability study. *Psychiatric Services, 73*(9), 1051–1055.

Manesh, N. E. (2017). Effectiveness of positive psychotherapy on stress in mothers of children with intellectual disability. *Journal of Exceptional Children, 17*(4), 5–14.

Morales-Sánchez, R., & Cabello-Medina, C. (2015). Integrating character in management: Virtues, character strengths, and competencies. *Business Ethics: A European Review, 24*, S156–S174.

Niemiec, R. M., Shogren, K. A., & Wehmeyer, M. L. (2017). Character strengths and intellectual and developmental disability: A strengths-based approach from positive psychology. *Education and Training in Autism and Developmental Disabilities, 52*(1), 13.

O'Driscoll, D. (2008). Psychotherapy and intellectual disability: A historical view. In T. Cottis & A. Alvarez (Eds.), *Intellectual disability, trauma and psychotherapy* (pp. 27–46). Routledge.

Park, N., & Peterson, C. (2008). Positive psychology and character strengths: Application to strengths-based school counseling. *Professional school counseling, 12*(2), 2156759X0801200214.

Peterson, C., & Seligman, M. E. (2004). *Character strengths and virtues: A handbook and classification*. Oxford University Press and American Psychological Association.

Raley, S. K., Shogren, K. A., & Cole, B. P. (2021). Positive psychology and education of students with disabilities: The way forward for assessment and intervention. *Advances in Neurodevelopmental Disorders, 5*, 11–20.

Rao, M. A., & Donaldson, S. I. (2015). Expanding opportunities for diversity in positive psychology: An examination of gender, race, and ethnicity. *Canadian Psychology, 56*(3), 271.

Rashid, T. (2015). Positive psychotherapy: A strength-based approach. *The Journal of Positive Psychology, 10*(1), 25–40.

Rashid, T. (2020). Positive psychotherapy. In *Encyclopedia of quality of life and well-being research* (pp. 1–8). Springer International Publishing.

Rashid, T., & Seligman, M. (2018). *Positive psychotherapy: Workbook*. Oxford University Press.

Rothman, D. J. (2017). *The Willowbrook wars: Bringing the mentally disabled into the community*. Routledge.

Schwartz, A. E., Caoili, A., Beasley, J. B., Kramer, J. M., & Kalb, L. G. (2022). Clinical applications of the VIA inventory of strengths with individuals with intellectual/developmental disabilities. *Journal of Positive Psychology, 18*, 439.

Seavey, M. (2012). Adapting Dialectical Behavior Therapy for clients with developmental disabilities and borderline personality disorder.

Seligman, M. E. P., & Adler, A. (2018). Positive education. *Global Happiness Policy Report*, 52–73.

Sheldon, K. M., & Schüler, J. (2011). Wanting, having, and needing: Integrating motive disposition theory and self-determination theory. *Journal of Personality and Social Psychology, 101*(5), 1106.

Shifrer, D., Callahan, R. M., & Muller, C. (2013). Equity or marginalization? The high school course-taking of students labeled with a learning disability. *American Educational Research Journal, 50*(4), 656–682.

Shogren, K. A., Niemiec, R. M., Tomasulo, D., & Khamsi, S. (2017a). Character strengths. In K. A. Shogren, M. L. Wehmeyer, & N. N. Singh (Eds.), *Handbook of positive psychology in intellectual and developmental disabilities: Translating research into practice* (pp. 189–199). Springer.

Shogren, K. A., Thompson, J. R., Wehmeyer, M. L., Seo, H., & Hagiwara, M. (2017b). Assessment in the application of positive psychology to intellectual and developmental disabilities. In *Handbook of positive psychology in intellectual and developmental disabilities: Translating research into practice* (pp. 37–46). Springer.

Slade, M. (2010). Mental illness and well-being: The central importance of positive psychology and recovery approaches. *BMC Health Services Research, 10*(1), 1–14.

Smieszek, M. (2019). Cinematherapy as a part of the education and therapy of people with intellectual disabilities, mental disorders and as a tool for personal development. *International Research Journal for Quality in Education, 6*(1), 30–34.

Smith, E. E. (2017). *The power of meaning*. Random House.

Szucs, A., Schau, C., Muscara, K., & Tomasulo, D. (2019). Character strength activation for people with intellectual and developmental disabilities using video feedback in groups. *Journal of Education and Learning, 8*(1), 12–20.

Szucs, A., Deebrah, M. R., & Hess, M. (2020). Hope at play: Mindfulness-informed group practices in action with people with intellectual and developmental disabilities before and during COVID-19. *International Journal of Arts Humanities and Social Sciences Studies, 5*(10).

Thompson Prout, H., & Browning, B. K. (2011). Psychotherapy with persons with intellectual disabilities: A review of effectiveness research. *Advances in Mental Health and Intellectual Disabilities, 5*(5), 53–59.

Tomasulo, D. J. (2014). Positive group psychotherapy modified for adults with intellectual disabilities. *Journal of Intellectual Disabilities, 18*(4), 337–350.

Tomasulo, D. J. (2015). *Action methods in group psychotherapy: Practical aspects*. Taylor & Francis.

Tomasulo, D. (2018). American snake pit: Hope, grit, and resilience in the wake of Willowbrook. .

Tomasulo, D., & Szucs, A. (2015). The ACTing cure: Evidence-based group treatment for people with intellectual disabilities. *Dramatherapy, 37*(2–3), 100–115.

Umucu, E., Lee, B., Genova, H. M., Chopik, W. J., Sung, C., Yasuoka, M., & Niemiec, R. M. (2022). Character strengths across disabilities: An international exploratory study and implications for positive psychiatry and psychology. *Frontiers in Psychiatry, 13*, 863977. https://doi.org/10.3389/fpsyt.2022.863977

Valldejuli, J. M. (2022). "Together we arrived and together we shall leave": The gouverneur parents association and the politics of race and disability in postwar New York. *Latino Studies, 20*(4), 428–454.

Whittle, E. L., Fisher, K. R., Reppermund, S., & Trollor, J. (2019). Access to mental health services: The experiences of people with intellectual disabilities. *Journal of Applied Research in Intellectual Disabilities, 32*(2), 368–379.

Zimbardo, P. (2011). *The Lucifer effect: How good people turn evil*. Random house.

Chapter 10
Spirituality in People with Intellectual/Developmental Disability

The Concepts

Spirituality is a significant, complex, universal part of the human experience, which varies in terms of beliefs, practices, rituals, and experiences of the transcendent, the sacred, or the divine (Niemiec et al., 2020; Peterson & Seligman, 2004). The most consistent definition from scientists is that spirituality is the search for, or communion with, the sacred (Pargament et al., 2013), with two-thirds of scientists using this definition (Kapuscinski & Masters, 2010). Some examples of the experience of the sacred include closeness with others, connection in nature, or oneness with a theist being, the transcendent, or all living beings (Davis et al., 2015). Spirituality involves a belief or understanding of a mystery in the universe that is beyond human understanding. Spirituality can be tapped and expressed through institutional religion and its rituals, beliefs, and community, therefore religion is one of many pathways for spirituality. As one of the 24 character strengths in the VIA Classification, spirituality is trait-like and refers to having coherent beliefs about one's place and purpose in the universe, about life meaning, and those beliefs shape one's relationships with others and the world (Peterson & Seligman, 2004).

In the co-edited book *Spirituality and Intellectual Disability*, editors Gaventa and Coulter (2001) discuss that while spirituality can be hidden or blocked by illness, disability, or other factors, it is not absent or lessened because conscious expression is lessened; they point out that consciousness may be a property of the brain but that spirituality is a property of the whole person—their subjective essence of being.

There exists the stereotype that spirituality for a person with IDD means only the most concrete of expressions, such as going to church, synagogue or mosque each week, praying before meals or bedtime, and sharing particular religious beliefs that have been passed down to them. Indeed, these are ways to connect with the sacred and tap into life meaning, however, we remind readers of the broader view of

R. M. Niemiec, D. Tomasulo, *Character Strengths and Abilities Within Disabilities*, Positive Psychology and Disability Series,
https://doi.org/10.1007/978-3-031-36294-1_10

spirituality as not only a character strength but also as a way of living one's life and interacting with others in a way that is fulfilling, meaningful, and connected.

Moreover, a look to the 24 character strengths reveals a wide range of spirituality tools for individuals with IDD (and those without). While any of the 24 character strengths can be viewed and expressed as spiritual, theologians, spiritual figures, and scientists in the broader field of spirituality would agree that several character strengths are clearly "spiritual" in nature (Niemiec et al., 2020). Examples of these include the character strengths of love, humility, gratitude, forgiveness, bravery, kindness, hope, fairness, awe/appreciation of beauty, zest, and as mentioned, the strength of spirituality (Carlisle & Tsang, 2013; Davis & Hook, 2014; Saroglou et al., 2008). Therefore, people with IDD have a myriad of character strengths within them to turn to experience and express their spirituality.

The reciprocal relationship between spirituality concepts/practices with character strengths concepts/practices has been articulated as two central pathways of integration—the grounding path and the sanctification path (Niemiec et al., 2020).

The grounding path: Character strengths → Spirituality → Wholeness.
The sanctification path: Spirituality → Character strengths → Wholeness.

The grounding path uses character strengths as a way to make spirituality—which can appear esoteric, ineffable, or vague—more accessible, layered, tangible, and meaningful. The sanctification path involves bringing aspects of the sacred and deep connection to strengths of character; in other words, to imbue one's best qualities with a significance and meaning that lends motivation power to one or more character strengths as they are tapped into or expressed. Both paths point toward greater wholeness, which refers to organizing life in a way that embracing one's brokenness, is life-affirming, and marked by breadth and depth (Pargament et al., 2016; Russo-Netzer, 2017).

The Science

Across the world, there largely remains a culture of exclusion, or at best tokenism, in terms of spiritual and communal integration of people with IDD (Raji & Gangemi, 2022). Spirituality is not an exceptionally well-understood area in the lives of people with IDD, especially in individuals with nonverbal autism (Hills et al., 2016). There has not been an abundance of studies examining spirituality in people with IDD, and the focus tends to be more as a reference to organized religion (Ault, 2010). Many of the studies and scholarship in the IDD literature tend to merge religiousness and spirituality and assume an integration for individuals. The larger literature has revealed that while there is overlap, the distinctions matter as spirituality has been shown to have more well-being and growth benefits than religiousness (Ivtzan et al., 2011); the largest meta-analysis to date ($N = 666{,}085$) also showed spirituality substantially outperformed religiosity for life satisfaction (Yaden et al., 2022).

Our focus in this section will reflect the common "merging" approach in order to stay true to the research studies, however, when available, distinctions will be drawn. We emphasize the lived experiences of people with IDD, the work on inclusiveness in spiritual communities, and spiritual practices.

In reviewing the literature on spirituality and people with IDD, Erik Carter (2021) observes several common themes:

1. Spirituality has relevance to the lives of individuals with IDD and their families.
2. Spirituality can have considerable importance.
3. Spirituality is experienced and expressed in very diverse ways.
4. Spirituality is rarely static.
5. Spirituality can be highly influential.
6. Spirituality can require planning and support (p. 425).

These themes reflect the substantial potential and importance of spirituality in the lives of people with IDD. This has been supported in interview studies in which people with IDD and autism share affirmation and acceptance of their disability as well as sharing the importance of faith and spirituality in their lives (e.g., Liu et al., 2014). Another review examining the role of spirituality in the lived experiences of people with disabilities and their parents highlighted that spirituality provides inner strength, peace, hope, and meaning, as well as promoting experiences of self-transformation through living with disability, becoming more mature and compassionate (Zhang & Rusch, 2005). Some of these themes were echoed in a mixed-methods approach by Rambow (2016) who found a significant positive relationship between spiritual well-being and quality of life among 50 people with IDD across gender and living situations; she followed this with a subset of 15 interviews that confirmed the results and revealed spirituality provided inner well-being, identity, connectedness, an opportunity to contribute, and a framework for life.

An interview study found there were different perceptions about the meaning of spirituality among adults with child-onset disabilities in comparison with those with adult-onset disabilities (Schulz, 2005). Although a small study of 12 individuals, the results revealed that spirituality was generally viewed as connecting/expressing through feelings and actions and that disability was a catalyst for spiritual awakening among adult-onset disabilities. Those with childhood onset disabilities noted spirituality was about connecting and expressing purpose/meaning in life and that disability was a vehicle to discover God's purpose.

Spiritual Community and Connections

While regular involvement in religious activities has been found to be much less common than other community activities such as eating out, shopping, and entertainment, the engagement with religious services is still high. A study of over 12,000 adults with IDD found that nearly half attended a religious service at least once in the previous month and 35% attended three or more times per month (Carter et al., 2015).

One study interviewed people with IDD and/or their carers and found that those living in a faith-based care service scored higher on a quality of life measure than those living in non-faith based care (Sango & Forrester-Jones, 2022). In addition, Sango and Forrester-Jones (2017) conducted a systematic review of IDD, spirituality, and social care services, ranging from 1990 to 2015, and found only five empirical articles that met their criteria for inclusion. The core themes they emphasized related to people with IDD understanding spiritual concepts, support and barriers in participating in activities, and practices relating to self-identity. Building from this research is the importance of social groups and belonging for people with IDD. Sango and Forrester-Jones (2018) found that a faith-based group of people with IDD had a larger social network of support than the individuals not in a faith-based group. Another study by these researchers emphasized the importance of spiritual care training and education to support people with IDD who are interested in such support (Sango & Forrester-Jones, 2019).

The importance of belonging is a recurring critical theme in the literature and as discussed in Chap. 3, the dynamics, processes, and strategies of people with IDD belonging in faith communities has been studied and championed by Erik Carter. Carter and his colleagues articulated 10 core themes of belonging for people with IDD into faith communities, arising from their in-depth interviews of individuals and their families. These included: being present, invited, welcomed, known, accepted, supported, cared for, befriended, needed, and loved (Carter, 2016; Carter et al., 2016). These themes offer not only researchers but practitioners, support professionals, families, and spiritual leaders a working road-map for connecting with people with IDD, including them, and helping them feel appreciated and integral to communities.

Spiritual Practices

There are a myriad of spiritual and religious practices of people with IDD that Carter and Boehm (2019) gathered in their research, for example, praying before meals, conversing with family members about spiritual issues, practicing a weekly day of rest, connecting with the divine through nature, and engaging in art, music, dance, or writing as a spiritual practice. Moreover, Carter and Boehm found that in asking 440 parents of children aged 13–21, that 10 spiritual/religious practices were engaged in on some kind of regular basis. They also found that 57% of parents report their child looking to their spirituality to provide meaning and purpose in their life. Another study found that prayer and positive religious coping strategies (and not negative religious coping strategies) were common among a group of 41 individuals with mild to moderate IDD (Shogren & Rye, 2005). Practical strategies for fostering spiritual development have been discussed in specific contexts for professionals, for example, Zhang (2010) offers interventions for teachers in special education.

Spirituality has been linked with other areas that have robust practices such as nature connection (Ferguson & Tamburello, 2015; Ryff, 2021) and mindfulness (Ivtzan, 2015; Lazaridou & Pentaris, 2016). Mindfulness research for people with IDD has received theoretical support (Shogren et al., 2017) and support in case studies (Singh et al., 2003). Preliminary research support for mindfulness practice for people with IDD has been found for boosting well-being and managing stress (Lake & MacHale, 2021), and improving confidence and reducing worries (Clyne et al., 2021). While traits of autism have been found to be associated with less pro-environmental behaviors (Taylor et al., 2021), there is a need for studies examining autism and IDD with nature connection as commissioned reports have found benefits for people with autism (Blakesley et al., 2013). Another study found that children with another neurodevelopmental disorder, ADHD, had reduced symptoms when they played in outdoor/green settings as opposed to human-built outdoor or indoor play settings (Taylor & Kuo, 2011). These lead to further questions of the potential value of nature and mindfulness for people with IDD and as potential mechanisms for experiencing and expressing spirituality.

The Practice

General Orientation

As practitioners address spirituality with people with IDD, a critical starting point is to understand one's own orientation and way of looking at the person. The way of looking will be influenced by the practitioner's or helper's own spirituality and the degree to which they have examined, denied, accepted, and worked with their own personal spirituality. Coulter (2001), in writing about and supporting spirituality in people with IDD, suggests three ways of looking at the person, which can be applied across the spectrum of ability and disability, across cultures, and across religious and spiritual beliefs. He explains the first way is to truly see the person as an individual human being, a spiritual being, not a client or case. This means to understand the spiritual ground of the person's existence, such as who they are, where they come from, who they love, what they value; it also involves looking with compassion and empathy. Coulter notes the second way of looking is to see the spirituality in common—that the person is a human being, a spiritual being, like oneself. In this view, the person's spirituality, existence, aliveness, and value as a person is seen, just as one sees these in oneself. "From this awareness of our own spirituality, we seek to recognize in the other person that which we know to be central to our own existence. Knowing what it means to me to be alive, I can then try to realize what it means for the other person to be alive" (p. 6). The third way of looking involves seeing in the other person the ground of all being, the transcendent, or divine. Coulter explains this third way of looking—in contrast to the first two—is quite uncommon and is largely out of our control and in the hands of the grace of God or a higher power.

Assessment

When considering the practical, it is useful to begin with assessment or at least an exploration of spirituality. The VIA Inventory of Strengths for Youth (i.e., VIA Youth Survey) measures the 24 character strengths in people ages 8–17, including the strength of spirituality (VIA Institute, 2023). The items on spirituality are the first in the scientific literature to assess spirituality in a secular way in young people while not colliding with spiritually oriented strengths such as forgiveness, kindness, or humility. While the VIA Youth Survey has been found to be generally inclusive and accessible for young people (Shogren et al., 2018) and support documents have been designed specifically for support people to guide (Shogren et al., 2015), the items need further improvement to be more concrete and accessible for people with IDD (Schwartz et al., 2022).

More than 20 years ago, Gaventa (2001) argued to the International Association for the Scientific Study of Intellectual Disability for "spiritual considerations" to be one of the five central dimensions of assessment of people with IDD, in addition to accepted dimensions of adaptive skills, psychological/emotional, physical health, and environmental. He articulated the various areas that would be involved in a spiritual assessment, including beliefs/meaning, vocation/calling, experience/emotion of the sacred or divine, courage/growth, rituals/practices, community, and where the individual looks for guidance/authority (from within, from outside themselves).

With any assessment measure or set of questions of spirituality for people with IDD, practitioners are encouraged to take an approach that is individualized to the person and emphasizes an active healthy spirituality. Gaventa positions this as a dimension of life and of growth; viewed as meaning, purpose, and coping; and viewed from a perspective of choice and self-determination (Gaventa, 2001).

Community

A number of approaches can be taken to support spiritual communities to grow from exclusion to inclusion to belonging for people with disabilities. This applies to churches, temples, mosques, synagogues, meditation/yoga groups, and other spiritual communities. In this regard, Carter (2021) suggests supporting individuals and families across seven central areas: reflecting, responding, inviting, preparing, supporting, befriending, and influencing.

1. Responding to the call found in sacred writings/scriptures, teaching, and practices to include others. In other words, practice what one preaches.
2. Reflecting on the community's own barriers, needs, and resources, and the perspectives of the individuals themselves, as opposed to following a prescriptive approach for inclusion.

3. Inviting people in a direct and potentially new way. Consistently sharing a message (newsletters, announcements, etc.) of inclusion, supports, and access, and partnering with disability agencies offers a clear message.
4. Preparing by building in support resources and a community mindset toward understanding and inclusion is a necessary action.
5. Supporting individuals that meet their unique needs, some of which might be more intensive and personalized, and may include new adaptations, support groups, or activities.
6. Befriending individuals by helping them to be known, needed, and loved, as opposed to solely existing in the building space. This may involve creating opportunities for individuals to have a role in the service or programming so that others in the community can get to know them.
7. Influencing those outside the community by communicating about the benefits and strength of the participation of individuals with disabilities and the impact on the community.

Practical Strategies

Next, we consider several practical strategies for potential spiritual expression. As each strategy is reviewed, studied, and practiced, we are reminded of what Gottlieb (2012) observed which is that any practice, whether it be meditation, prayer, service, etc., is only spiritual if it furthers the development of spiritual virtues. The following strategies are strong mechanisms—or potentialities—for advancing spiritual character strengths and virtues. Therefore, for each, we include the character strengths integration by someone with an IDD using the strategy.

Service/work/volunteering: What might an individual do to be part of their community and to contribute to the community, whether this be their neighborhood, city, workplace, school, or service community? What might the person share or do—from their own character strengths—in order to make the community better? Delila is a middle-aged woman with a developmental disability alongside a myriad of health concerns. She wanted to "give back" as an expression of her spirituality. She had the interest in singing as she frequently sang in the car, at home, and when she was with friends. She followed her passion and decided to go into a nursing home once per week to sing to the residents. She used her creativity to come up with a song arrangement, love of learning to memorize 50 songs, and her zest and kindness to deliver the music with passion and care to the audience. She filled herself with joy in this experience and the residents highly anticipated her events each week.

Community groups/faith communities: Advocate for oneself in the form of self-advocacy and in the form of advocacy by one's family, community members, and community leaders for not only inclusion but belonging in the spiritual community of one's choosing. Chris had a couple friends in a Buddhist meditation group that met once a week and he had felt a consistent sense of peace when he attended. He felt a longing for more and decided to use his bravery and honesty strengths to have a conversation with the meditation group's leader to advocate for his further involvement. The two brainstormed ideas and Chris resonated with an approach where, two times per month, he would invite the bell at the beginning and end of meditation and offer a short reading for the group to reflect on. He took his role seriously and played into his strengths of prudence and love in each offering of the bell and reading. Chris was overjoyed about this participation and received positive feedback from the members which led to steady community connectivity for Chris and the other members.

Mindfulness: The practice of bringing one's attention to the present moment with curiosity and openness can be applied to any aspect of life—conversations, working outdoors, washing dishes, eating supper, or playing with toys. Jade learned about an activity known as the mindful pause, which is two simple steps: take 15 seconds during the day to pause to breathe in and out, and conclude with a question to ask oneself, which of my character strengths might I use right now? (Niemiec, 2014). Jade practiced this approach two times a day, to feel more connected with herself and to feel more aligned with whatever she was doing. Often, the character strength that came up for her in the self-questioning was gratitude. She would then offer a "thank you" to wherever she was and whatever she was doing, for example, she thanked the sun, a swing she was on, the coffee she was drinking, or the electronic device she was playing on.

Nature connection: Spending time outdoors to purposefully connect with nature—planet Earth—is a common practice for many people to feel spiritually grounded and happy. Sade knew that walks in the woods in her backyard made her feel not only more refreshed but a sense of purpose and connection with something greater. She did short walks every morning by herself, and decided to involve a friend once a week so that this deeper connection could be shared with others. While on the walks, she readily felt her strength of appreciation of beauty rise up, as well as her love of learning to understand the different kinds of trees and small animals she encountered.

Consider the role of God, Higher Power, or a guiding force in one's life: Explore this with an open mind. Write about it, discuss it with others. For Judy, it was the route of discussion that was most important. She loved to share with zestful energy and a playful humor, and at the same time, she valued listening to others with an open, curious mind. She set up a plan once a week to have "spirituality discussions" with her relationship partner. They decided to create a ritual on Sunday evenings, so they could count on this practice at the same time each week. After a short period of quiet meditation, they took turns sharing and listening to one another about anything each considered to be "the spirit" moving in their life. Their topics ranged from sharing about a yoga practice, a scripture reading at church, a fun but meaningful spiritual meme seen online, to ways to make their relationship with one another more meaningful.

Daily life: For many people, spirituality is not only a trait-like characteristic but a default approach to return to in life experiences and the emotions, desires, struggles, and joys therein. To bring this important framing to life, we turn to practical suggestions in Gottlieb's (2012, pp. 7–8) seminal, scholarly book, *Spirituality: What It Is and Why It Matters*. He frames and infuses spirituality across different problems and vices people have and offers a simple strategy for facing, managing, or transcending the issue. For each example, we have added in one or more of the 24 character strengths (in *italics*), which seamlessly flow as spiritual pathways in each scenario. Many of these apply to the individual with disability themselves while others are more broad to others.

- If you are distracted or anxious, use *self-regulation* to turn off electronic devices and sit in silence.
- If you are angry, develop empathy (i.e., *social intelligence*, *love*) for those you are angry at; *honesty* toward your own struggles; and *bravery* to face grief or fear underlying your anger.
- If you are desirous of what others have, use *perspective* to see the limitless energy of the desires.
- If you overly pursue career or status and see emptiness or unfulfillment, turn to *love* to pursue the meaningful.
- If you are in despair because of a loss or negative transition, use your *social intelligence* and *bravery* to feel the depth of your sorrow and use *spirituality* and *appreciation of beauty* to find the simple goodness of life.
- If you are chronically ill, use your *honesty* to see your attachments and refusal to accept reality and *perseverance* to shape your mind to not make you worse.
- If people you love are ill, are self-destructive, or are tormenting you with their pain, use *forgiveness* and *perspective* to accept the inevitability of human suffering and *love* to love them and be a source of peace for them.
- If you are addicted to food, sex, or a substance, get *honest* about who you are, use *bravery* to make amends to those you have hurt, and *forgiveness* to let go and turn it over to a higher power.
- If you are grieving your child's disabilities, face the depth of your loss with *bravery* and *persevere* with *love* to value them for who they are and the *love*, *fairness*, *curiosity*, *hope*, and *gratitude* you can give them.
- If your relationship with God or larger forces in the universe has slipped into routine, use *zest* to reawaken your devotion and use *judgment* and *curiosity* to explore the meaning of each word of a familiar prayer.
- If you are hungry, look for someone to feed (*humility*, *kindness*); sad, look to cheer someone (*humor*, *hope*); need understanding, look to share it (*social intelligence*); needing care, go care for someone (*love*).

Future Directions

There is more that is unknown about the experience of spirituality in people with IDD than is known. Several studies in this chapter discuss aspects of the "lived experience" of spirituality for people with IDD. This leads to a number of research opportunities for mixed-methods studies to go deeper into types of meaning and purpose, transcendent experiences, and the myriad of ways to connect with the sacred. The integration of character strengths and spirituality for people with IDD is an unexplored area with potential for both basic and applied research. Intervention studies for people with IDD are few and far between, and even further for topics of spirituality and meaning, yet such studies would help us understand causal mechanisms and potential valued outcomes in this central area of human functioning.

Key Takeaways

- Spirituality is a universal part of the human experience, with the most common definition by scientists being that spirituality is the pursuit or communing with the sacred.
- Spirituality can be hidden or blocked by illness or disability but that does not mean it is absent or less or undervalued in people with IDD. Spirituality is the property of the whole person—their essence of being.
- Many of the 24 character strengths can be viewed as spiritual and thereby the VIA Classification provides pathways toward spirituality for each person, just as spirituality provides a pathway for a more sacred and meaningful expression of interior character strengths.
- While spirituality has been understudied in people with IDD, the literature is convincing in that spirituality is relevant, important, and often experienced and expressed by people with IDD and their families.
- Positive relationships between spirituality and well-being, identity, and connectedness have been found by researchers.
- Connecting in a spiritual community and feeling a sense of belonging therein is important for people with IDD, and frameworks have been developed to describe the process as well as ways the community can facilitate this belonging.
- Spirituality can be assessed and intervened upon in people with IDD.
- There are a number of spiritual practices that people with IDD report as beneficial, at home and in their communities.
- For a practice to be spiritual, it needs to further the development of spiritual virtues/character strengths.
- Practices along with case examples and spiritual character strengths uses can be viewed for service/work/volunteering, community groups/faith communities, mindfulness, nature connection, the role of God/Higher Power/guiding force, and multiple daily life vices, feelings, and struggles.

References

Ault, M. (2010). Inclusion of religion and spirituality in the special education literature. *The Journal of Special Education, 44*(3), 176189. https://doi.org/10.1177/0022466909336752

Blakesley, D., Rickinson, M., & Dillon, J. (2013). Engaging children on the autistic spectrum with the natural environment: Teacher insight study and evidence review. *Natural England Commissioned Reports*, NECR116.

Carlisle, R. D., & Tsang, J. A. (2013). The virtues: Gratitude and forgiveness. In K. I. Pargament, J. J. Exline, & J. W. Jones (Eds.), *APA handbook of psychology, religion, and spirituality (Vol. 1): Context, theory, and research* (pp. 423–437). American Psychological Association.

Carter, E. W. (2016). A place of belonging: Research at the intersection of faith and disability. *Review and Expositor, 113*(2), 167–180.

Carter, E. W. (2021). Spirituality and supports for individuals with intellectual and developmental disabilities and their families. In L. M. Glidden, L. Abbeduto, L. L. McIntyre, & M. J. Tassé (Eds.), *APA handbook of intellectual and developmental disabilities: Clinical and educational implications: Prevention, intervention, and treatment* (pp. 419–442). American Psychological Association. https://doi.org/10.1037/0000195-016

Carter, E. W., & Boehm, T. L. (2019). Religious and spiritual expressions of youth with intellectual and developmental disabilities. *Research and Practice for Persons With Severe Disabilities, 44*(1). https://doi.org/10.1177/15407969i9828082

Carter, E. W., Kleinert, H. L., LoBianco, T. E., Sheppard-Jones, K., Butler, L. N., & Tyree, M. S. (2015). Congregational participation of a national sample of adults with intellectual and developmental disabilities. *Intellectual and Developmental Disabilities, 53*(6), 381–393. https://doi.org/10.1352/1934955653.6.381

Carter, E. W., Biggs, E. E., & Boehm, T. L. (2016). Being present versus having a presence: Dimensions of belonging for young people with disabilities and their families. *Christian Education Journal, 13*(1), 127–146.

Clyne, C., Jackman, C., Tully, M., Coyle, D., & O'Reilly, G. (2021). We live in the moment—Experiences of people with intellectual disabilities and clinicians of computer-assisted mindfulness and relaxation. *British Journal of Learning Disabilities, 50*(3), 422–432. https://doi.org/10.1111/bld.12386

Coulter, D. L. (2001). Recognition of spirituality in health care: Personal and universal implications. *Journal of Religion, Disability & Health, 5*(2–3), 1–11.

Davis, D. E., & Hook, J. N. (2014). Humility, religion, and spirituality: An endpiece. *Journal of Psychology and Theology, 42*, 111–117. https://doi.org/10.1177/009164711404200112

Davis, D. E., Rice, K., Hook, J. N., Van Tongeren, D. R., DeBlaere, C., Choe, E., et al. (2015). Development of the sources of spirituality scale. *Journal of Counseling Psychology, 62*, 503. https://doi.org/10.1037/cou0000082

Ferguson, T. W., & Tamburello, J. A. (2015). The natural environment as a spiritual resource: A theory of regional variation in religious adherence. *Sociology of Religion, 76*(3), 295–314. https://doi.org/10.1093/socrel/srv029

Gaventa, W. C. (2001). Defining and assessing spirituality and spiritual supports: A rationale for inclusion in theory and practice. *Journal of Religion, Disability & Health, 5*(2–3), 29–48. https://doi.org/10.1300/J095v05n02_03

Gaventa, W. C., & Coulter, D. L. (2001). *Spirituality and intellectual disability: International perspectives on the effect of culture and religion on healing body, mind, and soul*. Haworth Press.

Gottlieb, R. S. (2012). *Spirituality: What it is and why it matters*. Oxford University Press.

Hills, K., Clapton, J., & Dorsett, P. (2016). Towards an understanding of spirituality in the context of nonverbal autism: A scoping review. *Journal of Disability & Religion, 20*(4), 265–290. https://doi.org/10.1080/23312521.2016.1244501

Ivtzan, I. (2015). *Awareness is freedom: The adventure of psychology and spirituality*. Changemakers Books.

Ivtzan, I., Chan, C. P. L., Gardner, H. E., & Prashar, K. (2011). Linking religion and spirituality with psychological wellbeing: Examining self actualisation, meaning in life, and personal growth initiative. *Journal of Religion and Health, 51*, 13–30.

Kapuscinski, A. N., & Masters, K. S. (2010). The current status of measures of spirituality: A critical review of scale development. *Psychology of Religion and Spirituality, 2*, 191–205. https://doi.org/10.1037/a0020498

Lake, S., & MacHale, R. (2021). Mindfulness matters: A pilot study of a mindfulness-based stress reduction group for adults with intellectual disabilities. *British Journal of Learning Disabilities, 50*(3), 412–421. https://doi.org/10.1111/bld.12435

Lazaridou, A., & Pentaris, P. (2016). Mindfulness and spirituality: Therapeutic perspectives. *Person-Centered & Experiential Psychotherapies, 15*(3), 235–244. https://doi.org/10.1080/14779757.2016.1180634

Liu, E. X., Carter, E. W., Boehm, T. L., Annandale, N., & Taylor, C. (2014). In their own words: The place of faith in the lives of young people with intellectual disability and autism. *Intellectual and Developmental Disabilities, 52*, 388–404. https://doi.org/10.1352/1934-9556-52.5.388

Niemiec, R. M. (2014). *Mindfulness and character strengths: A practical guide to flourishing*. Hogrefe.

Niemiec, R. M., Russo-Netzer, P., & Pargament, K. I. (2020). The decoding of the human spirit: A synergy of spirituality and character strengths toward wholeness. *Frontiers in Psychology, 11*, 2040. https://doi.org/10.3389/fpsyg.2020.02040

Pargament, K. I., Mahoney, A., Exline, J. J., Jones, J., & Shafranske, E. (2013). Envisioning an integrative paradigm for the psychology of religion and spirituality. In K. I. Pargament, J. Exline, & J. Jones (Eds.), *APA handbooks in psychology: APA handbook of psychology, religion, and spirituality: Vol 1, context, theory, and research* (pp. 3–20). American Psychological Association.

Pargament, K. I., Wong, S., & Exline, J. J. (2016). Wholeness and holiness: The spiritual dimension of eudaimonics. In J. Vittersø (Ed.), *Handbook of eudaimonic Well-being* (pp. 379–394). Springer.

Peterson, C., & Seligman, M. E. P. (2004). *Character strengths and virtues: A handbook and classification*. Oxford University Press/American Psychological Association.

Raji, O., & Gangemi, C. (2022). Intellectual disability. In C. C. H. Cook & A. Powell (Eds.), *Spirituality and psychiatry*. Cambridge University Press.

Rambow, T. (2016). The *relationship of spiritual wellbeing to quality of life in adults with intellectual and developmental disabilities* [Unpublished master's thesis]. Waterford Institute of Technology, Waterford, Ireland.

Russo-Netzer, P. (2017). Healing the divide through wholeness: Holding on to what makes us human. *International Journal of Existential Positive Psychology, 7*, 17.

Ryff, C. (2021). Spirituality and Well-being: Theory, science, and the nature connection. *Religions, 12*(11). https://doi.org/10.3390/rel12110914

Sango, P. N., & Forrester-Jones, R. (2017). Intellectual and developmental disabilities, spirituality and religion: A systematic review 1990–2015. *Journal of Disability & Religion, 21*(3), 280–295. https://doi.org/10.1080/23312521.2017.1317224

Sango, P. N., & Forrester-Jones, R. (2018). Spirituality and social networks of people with intellectual and developmental disability. *Journal of Intellectual & Developmental Disability, 43*(3), 274–228. https://doi.org/10.3109/13668250.2017.1310820

Sango, P. N., & Forrester-Jones, R. (2019). Spiritual care for people with intellectual and developmental disability: An exploratory study. *Journal of Intellectual & Developmental Disability, 44*(2), 150–160. https://doi.org/10.3109/13668250.2017.1350834

Sango, P. N., & Forrester-Jones, R. (2022). Spirituality and the quality of life of individuals with intellectual disability. *Journal of Long-Term Care*, 193–204. https://doi.org/10.31389/jltc.139

Saroglou, V., Buxant, C., & Tilquin, J. (2008). Positive emotions as leading to religion and spirituality. *Journal of Positive Psychology, 3*, 165–173. https://doi.org/10.1080/17439760801998737

Schulz, E. K. (2005). The meaning of spirituality for individuals with disabilities. *Disability and Rehabilitation, 27*(21), 1283–1295.

Schwartz, A. E., Caoili, A., Beasley, J. B., Kramer, J. M., & Kalb, L. G. (2022). Clinical applications of the VIA inventory of strengths with individuals with intellectual/developmental disabilities. *Journal of Positive Psychology*. https://doi.org/10.1080/17439760.2022.2036797

Shogren, K. A., & Rye, M. S. (2005). Religion and individuals with intellectual disabilities: An exploratory study of self-reported perspectives. *Journal of Religion, Disability & Health, 9*(1), 29–53. https://doi.org/10.1300/J095v09n01_03

Shogren, K. A., Wehmeyer, M. L., Forber-Pratt, A. J., & Palmer, S. B. (2015). *VIA inventory of strengths for youth (VIA-youth): Supplement for use when supporting youth with intellectual and developmental disabilities to complete the VIA-youth*. Kansas University Center on Developmental Disabilities. Document available here.

Shogren, K. A., Singh, N., Niemiec, R. M., & Wehmeyer, M. (2017). Character strengths and mindfulness. In M. Wehmeyer (Ed.), *Oxford handbooks online*. https://doi.org/10.1093/oxfordhb/9780199935291.013.77

Shogren, K. A., Shaw, L. A., Raley, S. K., Wehmeyer, M. L., Niemiec, R., & Adkins, M. (2018). Assessing character strengths in youth with intellectual disability: Reliability and factorial validity of the VIA-youth. *Intellectual and Developmental Disabilities, 56*(1), 13–29. https://doi.org/10.1352/1934-9556-56.1.13

Singh, N. N., Wahler, R. G., Adkins, A. D., & Myers, R. E. (2003). Soles of the feet: A mindfulness-based self-control intervention for aggression by an individual with mild mental retardation and mental illness. *Research in Developmental Disabilities, 24*(3), 158–169.

Taylor, A. F., & Kuo, F. E. (2011). Could exposure to everyday green spaces help treat ADHD? Evidence from children's play settings. *Applied Psychology: Health and Well-Being, 3*(3), 281–303. https://doi.org/10.1111/j.1758-0854.2011.01052.x

Taylor, E. C., Livingston, L. A., Callan, M. J., Hanel, P. H. P., & Shah, P. (2021). Do autistic traits predict pro-environmental attitudes and behaviors, and climate change belief? *Journal of Environmental Psychology, 76*. https://doi.org/10.1016/j.jenvp.2021.101648

VIA Institute (2023). *VIA assessments*. Available here: https://www.viacharacter.org/researchers/assessments

Yaden, D. B., Batz-Barbarich, C. L., Ng, V., Vaziri, H., Gladstone, J. N., Pawelski, J. O., & Tay, L. (2022). A meta-analysis of religion/spirituality and life satisfaction. *Journal of Happiness Studies, 23*, 4147–4163. https://doi.org/10.1007/s10902-022-00558-7

Zhang, K. C. (2010). Spirituality and disabilities: Implications for special education. *Intellectual and Developmental Disabilities, 48*(4), 299–302.

Zhang, D., & Rusch, E. R. (2005). The role of spirituality in living with disabilities. *Journal of Religion Disability & Health, 9*(1), 8398. https://doi.org/10.1300/J095v09n01_06

Appendices

Appendix 1: About the VIA Institute on Character

The mission of the VIA Institute on Character is short, yet complex: To advance the science and practice of character strengths.

Based in Cincinnati, Ohio, United States, the VIA Institute on Character is a non-profit organization dedicated to bringing the science of character strengths to the world. It creates and validates surveys of character and related constructs; conducts science to expand the breadth and depth of character strengths understanding, exploration, and application; supports hundreds of researchers per year by providing measurement tools and resources; offers a range of education materials (courses, tailored reports, videos, and practices); and develops practical strengths-based tools for individuals and professionals, such as counselors, managers, and educators.

Core to the VIA Institute is the belief that the rigorous, scientific pursuit to understand the range and dimensions of human goodness (e.g., character strengths) is the key to generating discoveries and strategies for improving the human experience that will enable and encourage the development and use of tools, practices, and methodologies which will fundamentally shift the trajectory of humankind toward the better.

Historically speaking, in the early 2000s, the VIA Institute supported pivotal work on the nature of positive character. A 3-year, 55-scientist investigation across the globe, led by Drs. Christopher Peterson and Martin Seligman, culminated in the landmark text *Character Strengths and Virtues: A Handbook and Classification*. The project also involved the creation of two valid and free measurement tools—the VIA Inventory of Strengths (colloquially known as the VIA Survey) for adults, and the VIA Youth Survey.

Around two decades later, by early 2023, there were over 30 million VIA Survey takers, 52 translations available for the adults, 28 translations available for youth,

R. M. Niemiec, D. Tomasulo, *Character Strengths and Abilities Within Disabilities*, Positive Psychology and Disability Series,
https://doi.org/10.1007/978-3-031-36294-1

over 900 research studies summarized on character strengths on the VIA site, and 195 countries (all) where the VIA Survey had been taken.

While "VIA" [vee-uh] once stood for "Values in Action" (Values in Action Inventory; Values in Action Institute, Values in Action Classification), the name was changed in 2006 to more precisely reflect the organization's work. VIA is a word in Latin that means "the path" or "the way" and serves as a bridging word. Indeed, the VIA character strengths have been shown scientifically to be *pathways* to greater well-being, better relationships and health, and to managing stress and adversity. At the same time, this work offers a *bridge* for science and practice and a bridge to help the general public lead more fulfilling lives.

Appendix 2: Character Strengths-Based IEPs & ISPs: Fact-Sheet

Character Strengths-Based IEPs & ISPs: Fact Sheet

IEPs: Supercharged with Character Strengths

- ✓ Include character strengths in every formal IEP to help with any difficulty/challenge.
- ✓ Character strengths are viewed as a *pathway* to help a student reach any goal and as support for any difficulty/challenge.
- ✓ This approach brings balance to the typical deficit-based, problem-focused approach.

ISPs: Individualized Strengths Plans

- ✓ For every student: An ISP focuses on the student's *character strengths*, **emphasizing** their highest, signature strengths.
- ✓ Collaborative approach involving the student, teachers, parents, & support profesionals.
- ✓ Focuses on character strengths goals to enhance well-being and manage stress/conflict/adversity.

Too often, teams discuss a student's strengths by saying things like, "What I like about this student is…." or "Jack likes baseball" or "Jill is good at math." These comments, while positive, can be hard to connect to in actionable ways OR they neglect to focus on who the student is - their core identity. IEP/ISP teams can reframe the discussion to character strengths: "What is best about this student? What makes them shine?"

For example, for a student who struggles in math, how do they use their character strengths well with other subjects and situations? Do they use curiosity to explore the subject? Do they show prudence to plan out their study approach? Do they prefer to work well in a group (teamwork)? Strengths-based IEPs/ISPs aim to bring character strengths into each of the skill sets and performance goals.

Tips for how teachers can learn to be "character strengths-based" with IEPs/ISPs:

Use the **VIA Survey & VIA Youth Survey** to identify signature strengths and the	Practice *strengths-spotting* with every student in class and within every **IEP meeting**. Encourage self-	Weave character strengths into **IEP goals** to tap into core identity & the	Expanding **IEP templates** to include character strengths as tools & pathways for

Examples of Character Strength IEPs and ISPs

IEP goal, traditional example: Sarah will show understanding of another's feelings.

IEP, supercharged with character strengths: Sarah will use her strengths of love and curiosity to show understanding of another's feelings. Teacher will practice strength-spotting when Sarah uses questions to understand feelings.

ISP (individualized strengths plan): Sarah will use her signature strengths each day in the classroom. She'll use her strength of *curiosity* to ask her peers one new question per day. She'll use her *bravery* to face her discomfort in handling schedule changes. When Sarah feels overwhelmed, she will use her strength of *prudence* to plan the task at hand with smaller steps.

- Sarah's parents/teacher will reinforce her signature strengths & will practice strengths-spotting in Sarah at home and in the classroom.

VIA INSTITUTE ON CHARACTER

Ryan M. Niemiec, PsyD, Chief Science & Education Officer, VIA Institute on Character

Index

R. M. Niemiec, D. Tomasulo, *Character Strengths and Abilities Within Disabilities*, Positive Psychology and Disability Series,
https://doi.org/10.1007/978-3-031-36294-1

W

Z

The manufacturer's authorised representative in the EU is Springer Nature Customer Service Centre GmbH, Europaplatz 3, 69115 Heidelberg, Germany. If you have any concerns regarding our products, please contact ProductSafety@springernature.com

Printed and bound by CPI Group (UK) Ltd, Croydon, CR0 4YY

28/09/2026

02224070-0003